T0226849

Wound Management

Editor

MARIJE RISSELADA

VETERINARY CLINICS OF NORTH AMERICA: SMALL ANIMAL PRACTICE

www.vetsmall.theclinics.com

November 2017 • Volume 47 • Number 6

ELSEVIER

1600 John F. Kennedy Boulevard • Suite 1800 • Philadelphia, Pennsylvania, 19103-2899
http://www.vetsmall.theclinics.com

VETERINARY CLINICS OF NORTH AMERICA: SMALL ANIMAL PRACTICE Volume 47, Number 6
November 2017 ISSN 0195-5616, ISBN-13: 978-0-323-54909-7

Editor: Colleen Dietzler
Developmental Editor: Meredith Madeira

Veterinary Clinics of North America: Small Animal Practice (ISSN 0195-5616) is published bimonthly by Elsevier Inc., 360 Park Avenue South, New York, NY 10010-1710. Months of issue are January, March, May, July, September, and November. Business and Editorial Offices: 1600 John F. Kennedy Blvd., Ste. 1800, Philadelphia, PA 19103-2899. Customer Service Office: 3251 Riverport Lane, Maryland Heights, MO 63043. Periodicals postage paid at New York, NY and additional mailing offices. Subscription prices are $319.00 per year (domestic individuals), $598.00 per year (domestic institutions), $100.00 per year (domestic students/residents), $422.00 per year (Canadian individuals), $743.00 per year (Canadian institutions), $469.00 per year (international individuals), $743.00 per year (international institutions), and $220.00 per year (international and Canadian students/residents). To receive student/resident rate, orders must be accompanied by name of affiliated institution, date of term, and the *signature* of program/residency coordinator on institution letterhead. Orders will be billed at individual rate until proof of status is received. Foreign air speed delivery is included in all *Clinics* subscription prices. All prices are subject to change without notice. **POSTMASTER:** Send address changes to *Veterinary Clinics of North America: Small Animal Practice*, Elsevier Health Sciences Division, Subscription Customer Service, 3251 Riverport Lane, Maryland Heights, MO 63043. Customer Service (orders, claims, online, change of address): Elsevier Periodicals Customer Service, Elsevier Health Sciences Division Subscription **Customer Service 3251 Riverport Lane Maryland Heights, MO 63043. Tel: 1-800-654-2452 (U.S. and Canada); 314-447-8871 (outside U.S. and Canada). Fax: 314-447-8029. E-mail: journalscustomerservice-usa@elsevier.com (for print support); journalsonlinesupport-usa@elsevier.com (for online support).**

Reprints. For copies of 100 or more of articles in this publication, please contact the Commercial Reprints Department, Elsevier Inc., 360 Park Avenue South, New York, NY 10010-1710. Tel.: 212-633-3874; Fax: 212-633-3820; E-mail: reprints@elsevier.com.

Veterinary Clinics of North America: Small Animal Practice is also published in Japanese by Inter Zoo Publishing Co., Ltd., Aoyama Crystal-Bldg 5F, 3-5-12 Kitaaoyama, Minato-ku, Tokyo 107-0061, Japan.

Veterinary Clinics of North America: Small Animal Practice is covered in *Current Contents/Agriculture, Biology and Environmental Sciences, Science Citation Index, ASCA, MEDLINE/PubMed (Index Medicus), Excerpta Medica, and BIOSIS.*

Contributors

EDITOR

MARIJE RISSELADA, DVM, PhD
Diplomate, European College of Veterinary Surgeons; Diplomate, American College of Veterinary Surgeons-Small Animal; Formerly, Assistant Professor, Small Animal Soft Tissue and Oncologic Surgery, Department of Clinical Sciences, North Carolina State University, College of Veterinary Medicine, Raleigh, North Carolina, USA; Currently, Assistant Professor, Small Animal Surgery, Department of Veterinary Clinical Sciences, College of Veterinary Medicine, Purdue University, West Lafayette, Indiana, USA

AUTHORS

LAURA C. CUDDY, MVB, MS
Diplomate, American College of Veterinary Surgeons; Diplomate, European College of Veterinary Surgeons; Diplomate, American College of Veterinary Sports Medicine and Rehabilitation; Staff Surgeon, Vets Now 24/7 Emergency and Specialty Hospital, Manchester, United Kingdom; Director, Veterinary Specialists, Summerhill, County Meath, Ireland

CHRISTINE A. CULLER, DVM, MS
Diplomate, American College of Veterinary Emergency and Critical Care; Fellow, Extracorporeal Therapy, Department of Clinical Sciences, North Carolina State University, College of Veterinary Medicine, Raleigh, North Carolina, USA

HILDE DE ROOSTER, DVM, MVM, PhD
Diplomate, European College of Veterinary Surgeons; Associate Professor, Small Animal Department, Faculty of Veterinary Medicine, Ghent University, Merelbeke, Belgium

NAUSIKAA DEVRIENDT, DVM
Research Associate, Small Animal Department, Faculty of Veterinary Medicine, Ghent University, Merelbeke, Belgium

TRACY GIEGER, DVM
Clinical Assistant Professor, Department of Clinical Sciences, North Carolina State University, College of Veterinary Medicine, Raleigh, North Carolina, USA

KELLEY THIEMAN MANKIN, DVM, MS
Diplomate, American College of Veterinary Surgeons-Small Animal; Assistant Professor, Department of Small Animal Clinical Sciences, College of Veterinary Medicine and Biomedical Sciences, Texas A&M University, College Station, Texas, USA

MICHAEL NOLAN, DVM, PhD
Assistant Professor, Department of Clinical Sciences, North Carolina State University, College of Veterinary Medicine, Raleigh, North Carolina, USA

MARIJE RISSELADA, DVM, PhD
Diplomate, European College of Veterinary Surgeons; Diplomate, American College of Veterinary Surgeons-Small Animal; Formerly, Assistant Professor, Small Animal Soft Tissue and Oncologic Surgery, Department of Clinical Sciences, North Carolina State University, College of Veterinary Medicine, Raleigh, North Carolina, USA; Currently, Assistant Professor, Small Animal Surgery, Department of Veterinary Clinical Sciences, College of Veterinary Medicine, Purdue University, West Lafayette, Indiana, USA

VALERY F. SCHARF, DVM, MS
Diplomate, American College of Veterinary Surgeons; Assistant Professor, Small Animal Soft Tissue Surgery, Department of Clinical Sciences, North Carolina State University, College of Veterinary Medicine, Raleigh, North Carolina, USA

BRYDEN J. STANLEY, BVMS, MACVSc, MVetSc
Diplomate, American College of Veterinary Surgeons; Section Chief, Surgery, College of Veterinary Medicine, Michigan State University, East Lansing, Michigan, USA

ELIZABETH THOMPSON, DVM
Surgery, North Carolina State University, College of Veterinary Medicine, Raleigh, North Carolina, USA

ALESSIO VIGANI, DVM, PhD
Diplomate, American College of Veterinary Emergency and Critical Care; Diplomate, American College of Veterinary Anesthesia and Analgesia; Clinical Assistant Professor, ECC and Extracorporeal Therapy, Department of Clinical Sciences, North Carolina State University, College of Veterinary Medicine, Raleigh, North Carolina, USA

Contents

> When traumatic wounds are quickly and accurately treated, morbidity and costs can be significantly decreased. Several factors, such as time delay between injury and treatment, the degree of contamination, extension and depth of the wound, and the mechanism of injury, influence the treatment and prognosis and stress the importance of a patient-specific approach. Although all traumatic wounds are contaminated, antibiotic therapy is seldom required if correct wound management is installed.

> Most body wall injuries in small animals are caused by bite wounds or vehicular trauma. Penetrating gunshot wounds are less common. Bite wounds are characterized by massive trauma to the body wall with associated defects, but fewer internal injuries, whereas gunshot wounds are associated with a high number of internal injuries. Vehicular accident injuries are caused by blunt force trauma and can lead to both body wall defects and internal organ damage. Impalement injuries are rare and are typically associated with internal damage. Exploratory surgery, herniorrhaphy, and aggressive wound management are recommended in the treatment of these injuries.

> Management of severe burn injury (SBI) requires prompt, complex, and aggressive care. Despite major advances in the management of SBI, including patient-targeted resuscitation, management of inhalation injuries, specific nutritional support, enhanced wound therapy, and infection control, the consequences of SBI often result in complex, multiorgan metabolic changes. Consensus guidelines and clinical evidence regarding specific management of small animal burn patients are lacking. This article reviews updated therapeutic consideration for the systemic and local management of SBI that are proven effective to optimize outcomes in human burn patients and may translate to small animal patients.

> Radiation therapy (RT) is an essential component for management of many cancers. Veterinary health care professionals must counsel owners about

the potential side effects of RT, the anticipated management plan, and associated costs. For most veterinary patients treated with RT, acute radiation side effects are mild; however, careful radiation treatment planning and appropriate management of acute side effects are essential to try to prevent chronic sequelae and the need for ongoing wound care. This article reviews acute and late side effects to the skin and their management.

The importance of initial wound classification and daily reevaluation of wound stage cannot be understated. Products available to enhance healing are categorized based on the stage of wound healing to which they exert their effects. After patient stability has been verified, thorough debridement is critical to create an environment conducive for healing. The wound environment of acute and chronic wounds differs greatly, often requiring different management approaches.

 Video content accompanies this article at http://www.vetsmall.theclinics.com.

Open wounds are regularly addressed in veterinary medicine and can be challenging to manage, especially when there is significant loss of full-thickness skin. Traditional wound dressings are being replaced by modern synthetic materials, biologic wound dressings, and mechanical technologies to augment healing. Negative pressure wound therapy (NPWT) is one of the most successful mechanical adjuncts to wound healing. Experience with NPWT in veterinary medicine is not as extensive as in human medicine, but reports have been positive. This modality may become an invaluable adjunct to wound management and other surgical applications in both large and small animals.

Wounds are often addressed by primary or delayed primary closure. Although many skin wounds could go on to heal by second intention, this results in a less cosmetic outcome, takes longer, and in the long run, is often more expensive. As a general rule, the simplest method of wound closure that is likely to succeed should be chosen. If tension is present at the wound edges, wound dehiscence is likely to occur. Using specific techniques to relieve tension on wound edges and recruiting local flaps from neighboring regions are useful ways to achieve wound closure.

Axial pattern flaps are based on a direct cutaneous artery and vein supplying a segment of skin. They provide a large, robust option for large wound closure. Many different axial pattern flaps have been described to provide options for closure of wounds located from the nose to the tail. All axial pattern flaps require good surgical technique and careful attention to detail while developing the flap.

Valery F. Scharf

Skin grafts and free skin flaps are useful options for closure of wounds in which primary closure or use of traditional skin flaps is not feasible. Grafts are classified by their morphology and host-donor relationship. Free skin flaps with microvascular anastomoses are developed from previously described axial pattern flaps and have the added advantage of reestablishing robust vascular supply to the flap, but require specialized equipment and a high degree of technical expertise. Despite intensive perioperative care and the risk of graft or flap failure, skin grafts and free skin flaps can serve as rewarding methods of closing difficult wounds.

VETERINARY CLINICS OF NORTH AMERICA: SMALL ANIMAL PRACTICE

RELATED INTEREST

Veterinary Clinics: Small Animal Practice
September 2015, Volume 45, Issue 5
Perioperative Care
Lori S. Waddell, *Editor*
Available at: http://www.vetsmall.theclinics.com

THE CLINICS ARE NOW AVAILABLE ONLINE!
Access your subscription at:
www.theclinics.com

Preface

Wound Management

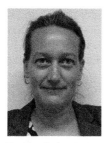

Marije Risselada, DVM, PhD
Editor

Wound management in *Veterinary Clinics of North America: Small Animal Practice* is an ever-evolving field with new techniques and products continually being developed at the same time some classical options persist. The authors of this issue introduce and establish that the wide variety of aspects of wound management, ranging from initial evaluation and treatment of patients, to the treatment of chronic wounds, and specific types of wounds, as well as options that exist to close large and/or difficult defects.

The groundwork for the successful treatment of patients with extensive wounds and the wounds themselves is laid with the first presentation. In the first article, "Initial Management of Traumatic Wounds," decision-making options, techniques, and products are discussed for first-line wound management.

In some instances, the external extent of the wound might belie its significance, and associated injuries could be life threatening. One such example is perforating wounds, and the diagnostic evaluation, management, and prognosis of these injuries are discussed in the second article, "Perforating Cervical, Thoracic, and Abdominal Wounds."

Burn wounds may have extensive systemic effects, particularly when large surface areas are involved. The third article, "Systemic and Local Management of Burn Wounds," discusses the management of burn wounds as well as their systemic implications and management.

As radiation therapy becomes more widely available, the veterinary profession may see more side effects following treatment. One such side effect is to the skin within the radiation field. The article entitled, "Management of Radiation Side Effects to the Skin," expands on the cause and management of radiation-induced skin damage.

The main goal of the next two articles is open wound management. The first of these articles summarizes management options and products available for open wound management that have been classically available and are still used currently, with the exception of negative pressure wound therapy (NPWT) ("Debridement Techniques

Vet Clin Small Anim 47 (2017) ix–x
http://dx.doi.org/10.1016/j.cvsm.2017.08.015
0195-5616/17/© 2017 Published by Elsevier Inc.

and Non–Negative Pressure Wound Therapy Wound Management"). One of the biggest advances in more recent years has been the introduction of NPWT, which has quickly become a mainstay in the management of large skin defects and complicated wounds. The article, "Negative Pressure Wound Therapy," explores the underlying theory and practical application of NPWT.

The final three articles explore and summarize strategies for closing difficult and large skin defects and wounds. The article, "Wound Closure, Tension-Relieving Techniques, and Local Flaps," starts with local management of difficult-to-close wounds, whereas the article, "Axial Pattern Flaps," summarizes techniques that can be used to close large defects or defects in locations where additional bulk or strength is needed. Last, the article, "Free Grafts and Microvascular Anastomoses," explores advanced surgical techniques for sites that cannot be repaired with local techniques or axial pattern flaps.

I would like to thank the authors who contributed to this issue and hope that this work will serve as a useful and oft-used resource when thinking about treatment options for difficult wounds.

Marije Risselada, DVM, PhD
Department of Veterinary Clinical Sciences
College of Veterinary Medicine
Purdue University
Lynn Hall, 625 Harrison Street
West Lafayette, IN 47907, USA

E-mail address:
mrissela@purdue.edu

Initial Management of Traumatic Wounds

Nausikaa Devriendt, DVM, Hilde de Rooster, DVM, MVM, PhD*

KEYWORDS

- Traumatic wounds • Wound management • Dog • Cat

KEY POINTS

- When traumatic wounds are quickly and accurately treated, morbidity and costs can be significantly decreased.
- Several factors, such as time delay between injury and treatment, the degree of contamination, extension and depth of the wound, and the mechanism of injury, influence the treatment and prognosis and stress the importance of a patient-specific approach.
- Although all traumatic wounds are contaminated, antibiotic therapy is seldom required if correct wound management is installed.

INTRODUCTION

Intact skin forms a protective barrier to the external environment. Damage to the skin allows bacteria to enter, causing inflammation and local or systemic infection.[1]

Management Goals

The primary goal of wound management is to achieve healing as quickly as possible to minimize pain, prevent infection, and restore normal function.[1,2] Inflammation, infection, or debris may delay or prevent wound healing and should therefore be addressed adequately.[3,4] Wound management consists of several steps that consistently need to be followed to ensure optimal wound healing and to minimize morbidity (**Fig. 1**).

INITIAL PATIENT ASSESSMENT

- Take a thorough history from the owner or eyewitness (**Box 1**).[5]

Disclosure Statement: The authors have nothing to disclose.
Small Animal Department, Faculty of Veterinary Medicine, Ghent University, Salisburylaan 133, Merelbeke 9820, Belgium
* Corresponding author.
E-mail address: hilde.derooster@ugent.be

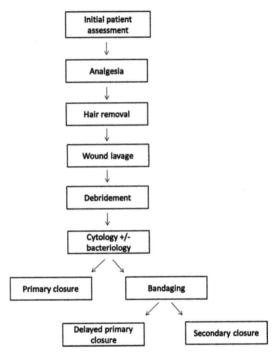

Fig. 1. Flow chart of wound management of acute traumatic wounds.

- Perform a complete physical examination, including a complete orthopedic and neurologic examination.[5–7]
- Triage and resuscitation, if applicable, should proceed wound management.[6,8]
- Analgesics should be administered before manipulation of the injured animal.[6,9]
- Cover wound surface to decrease likelihood of contamination and/or infection and avoid further injury in anticipation of definitive wound management.[5,6]

Box 1
Key points in the history of wounds influencing the possibility of infection and the prospect of healing

The cause of the injury[7,10,11]

The degree of injury[7,10,11]

Time elapsed from the injury[7,10,11]

Further insults since the injury[5]

Likelihood of contamination from the surrounding environment[5]

Previous installed treatment by the owner or referring veterinarian[5]

Probability of retained foreign bodies[7]

WOUND ASSESSMENT

Once the patient is clinically stable, a thorough wound assessment should be performed (**Box 2**). It is imperative to assess wounds on extremities through a full range of motion.[4] If necessary, animals should be sedated or placed under general anesthesia.[5]

Bacteria in the wound might not only come from the endogenous skin microflora or from an exogenous source during trauma, but also come from the examiner's hands.[10] As a consequence, general hygiene is very important, such as washing hands and wearing gloves.

Bleeding can be obvious or hidden and can trigger hypovolemic shock.[8,11] Arterial damage dictates early exploration and repair or ligation of the ruptured vessel; blind clamping is not recommended, because it may be associated with inadvertent damage to other structures.[9] Venous hemorrhage can usually be adequately controlled by direct pressure, even if veins are large.[8] Generalized oozing from capillaries should not be underestimated and can cause significant blood loss if the injury is extensive.[8] During exploration of the wound, further damage to structures should be avoided.[7]

CLASSIFICATION OF TRAUMATIC WOUNDS

Traumatic wounds can be classified based on factors that affect wound healing and management (**Box 3**). Nevertheless, wound management needs to be tailored to the individual wound in the individual patient.[12]

Time Delay Between Injury and Treatment

Delay in treatment is associated with proliferation and tissue invasion by bacteria and infection.[13] The so-called golden period is the time necessary for bacteria to reach a level of more than 10^5 per gram of tissue (or per milliliter of exudate).[13,14] This period is variable in time and depends on the initial amount of bacteria in the wound, their virulence, local and systemic defense mechanisms of the host,[13,15,16] and the vascularity of the tissue.[7] In general, the accepted interval from injury to wound treatment is up to 6 hours,[1,7] although some researchers claim it is only 3 hours.[13] In any case, delay in treatment of acute wounds should be avoided. Subacute wounds (>6 hours) are always considered contaminated, unless measures were taken to clean them regularly and protective dressings were applied.[1]

Degree of Contamination

All traumatic wounds are contaminated to a certain level, even if only by normal skin flora[15,17]; however, not all wounds are initially infected.[14] It is imperative to distinguish

---

Box 2
Important aspects of wound assessment

Location[4,7,10]

Dimensions[4,7]

Involvement of underlying tissues[4,7,10]

Involvement of thoracic or abdominal cavity[4,7]

Functional status of surrounding structures[4,7,10]

Presence of foreign body[7]

Associated contaminants[4]

Box 3
Major parameters in classification of acute traumatic wounds

Time delay

Less than 6 h versus greater than 6 h
  Amount and type of bacteria
  Tissue viability
  Host defenses

Degree of contamination

Contaminated versus infected
  Time delay
    Amount and type of bacteria
    Tissue viability
    Host defenses
  ± Foreign bodies
  ± Penetrating injury

Depth and extension

Tissue viability

Mechanism of injury

Sharp versus blunt

Low versus high velocity

---

wound contamination from wound infection; in the latter, microorganisms not only replicate but also cause subsequent host injury as well.[18] Not only the amount and type of bacteria but also the time delay to treatment dictate the relative probability of infection.[19]

Careful examination of the wound is recommended if there is any chance of retained foreign bodies, because they increase the risk of an inflammatory response and subsequent infection and abscess formation. Furthermore, they might migrate, cause persistent pain, or impair mechanical function.[7] Penetrating foreign bodies should never be removed before surgery, because their presence might prevent ruptured blood vessels from bleeding.[20] Penetrating traumas to the thoracic or abdominal cavity require a specific approach (please see Marije Risselada's article, "Perforating Cervical, Thoracic, and Abdominal Wounds," in this issue for more information). Medical imaging might be required to detect the presence of foreign bodies or to evaluate damage to surrounding tissues.[7,9,11,21]

The degree of contamination at the time of treatment is an important feature, which will determine if a wound has to be treated as an open wound to decrease bioburden or if primary closure is possible. Heavy bacterial bioburden negatively impacts wound healing by increasing the metabolic requirements of the patient, by stimulating a proinflammatory environment, and by the negative effects of cytokines secreted by bacteria.[22] Wounds that are treated within the golden period can usually be converted to clean or clean-contaminated wounds.[1,5,19] Wounds with devitalized tissue or perforated viscera or more chronic traumatic wounds with clinically overt infection are classified as dirty wounds.[17]

Extension and Depth of Wound

Deep lacerations with devitalized tissue are more prone to infection than superficial abrasions. They cause destruction of soft tissues with variable amounts of devitalization.[21,23] Superficial wounds are generally easily converted to clean wounds, whereas extensive or deep wounds often need repeated cleaning before definitive treatment can be performed.[1]

Mechanism of Injury

The cause of the injury influences the wound's susceptibility to infection.

Penetrating trauma results in the destruction of soft tissues with variable amounts of underlying tendon, nerve, bone, and vascular disruption.[21]

Bite wounds may appear as small puncture wounds externally, despite large internal lacerations.[24] Likewise, blunt trauma, crush wounds, and degloving and avulsion injuries can result in large areas of tissue destruction, the extent of which is not always obvious at first sight.[21] With these types of wounds, the tissues absorb a large amount of energy, reducing the blood flow to the wound edges and decreasing defense mechanisms.[23] Shearing or degloving injuries cause significant devascularization with subsequent necrosis.[1] Crush injuries cause immediate cell death and damage to the underlying blood supply.[1]

High-velocity wounds (such as gunshots) cause a great deal of damage in deeper tissues because of the dissipation of kinetic energy. Furthermore, behind the bullet there is a sucking action that deposits dirt and hair in the wound. Together with ischemia, this contamination provides an ideal culture medium for anaerobic bacteria.[8]

HAIR REMOVAL

Hair removal prevents hair from becoming entangled or falling in the wound; it helps to clean the surroundings of the wound, and it prevents interference with the application of dressings.[5,25] Hair should be clipped from a wide area around the wound edges.[5] Especially in patients with bite wounds, wide shaving might reveal additional puncture wounds that were hidden under fur.[6]

Damage to the skin should be prevented during clipping to avoid skin contamination from bacteria located in the hair follicles. To avoid hair entering the wound during the process of shaving, either sterile lubricant or sterile, moist gauze sponges should cover the wound bed and hair should be clipped from the wound edges toward the periphery.[5,26] After clipping, hair and sponges are removed and lubricant is subsequently rinsed away.[5]

LAVAGE

Wound irrigation is an important aspect of wound management; it helps to decrease bacterial contamination and physically removes foreign bodies, debris, and any other loose material from the wound.[27–29] Cleaning of the clipped area is beneficial, but inadvertent spillage of antiseptics into the wound should be avoided because it causes an inflammatory response, increasing the wound's susceptibility to bacterial infection.[30,31]

In order to remove the wound debris, the force of the irrigation stream has to be greater than the adhesion forces holding the debris to the wound surface.[28] A pressure of 8 to 12 psi is required to dislodge bacteria from the wound surface and reduce the risk of infection.[28,32] Nevertheless, higher pressures can cause dispersion of bacteria into the wound, impair wound defenses, and inadvertently cause loose fascial planes to separate.[33,34]

An 18-gauge needle attached to a 20-mL syringe or a 19-gauge needle attached to a 30-mL syringe delivers a stream to the surface at the optimal pressure.[28,35] The further the irrigant is from the wound, the lower the impact pressure exerted on the tissues.[36] Ideally, lavage is applied at an oblique angle to effectively dislodge debris and bacteria.[34] Connection of the needle and syringe via a "3-way" connector to an infusion bag with saline is an easy way to use this.[28] Although lavage diminishes bacterial counts in all wounds, only pulsatile jet lavage causes a significant reduction of bacteria and removes necrotic tissue and foreign particles from wounds.[21,27,37,38] The main disadvantage of pulsatile jet lavage is that it may disseminate bacteria in the environment because of the formation of an aerosol during application.[29] Although many studies have been done, no optimal irrigation technique has been identified so far.[39] Moreover, one study showed that different persons using the same irrigation technique apply different amounts of pressure to the wound.[40] The optimal pressure for wound irrigation depends on the wound characteristics, such as the size of particles in the wound, the amount of contamination, and the type of injury (stab wound vs shearing injury).[23,39]

Thorough lavage can be done with isotonic solutions such as normal saline (0.9%) or Ringer solution.[5] There is no significant advantage in using an antimicrobial or surfactant as an irrigant over normal saline in preventing wound infection.[41] Although antiseptic solutions can reduce the bacterial concentration on intact skin, they appear cytotoxic to the wound bed and hinder wound defense mechanisms. Although tap water has been shown to be a safe, efficacious, and cost-effective alternative to sterile saline in human medicine,[42,43] it is shown to cause considerable fibroblast injury in dogs[44] and, as a consequence, delays the healing process.

The volume of irrigation should be adjusted to the wound characteristics and degree of contamination.[21] The entire wound surface should be irrigated and that may require pulling open the wound edges and flaps for exposure.[45] Large volumes, with a minimum of 150 to 200 mL, should be delivered to the wound,[32,46] and ideally, the fluid should be body-warm.[47]

DEBRIDEMENT

Debridement involves the removal of adherent, nonviable, contaminated, or necrotic tissue from the wound, because this is the ideal environment for bacterial growth and because this interferes with wound healing.[5,21,29,48–50] Furthermore, the presence of avascular or necrotic tissue within a wound prevents penetration of antimicrobials into the tissue regardless of its route of administration.[51] It is important not only to debride the wound bed but also to debride the wound edges and periwound skin.[29]

Although debridement is often only needed once in acute wounds,[50] subsequent debridement may be necessary when there is an inability to accurately predict the amount of nonviable tissue and extent of debridement required during initial assessment, or if the infectious bioburden is high.[5,21,48] Although viability of skin is usually easy to judge, demarcation of muscle is not always that apparent.[48] Moreover, in high-velocity injuries, the magnitude of tissue injury is extensive and difficult to ascertain soon after injury. In those cases, foreign bodies should be removed, vascular damage should be ruled out, and the development of compartment syndrome should be precluded.[48]

Different types of wound debridement exist, which are discussed in Elizabeth Thompson's article, "Debridement Techniques and Non–Negative Pressure Wound Therapy Wound Management," in this issue.

CYTOLOGY AND BACTERIOLOGY

After lavage and debridement, samples for cytology and bacteriology are taken, ideally before topical or systemic antimicrobial treatment is initiated.[6,52] Cytology can help to differentiate between contamination by commensals and real pathogens. The former will be found extracellularly in smears with few inflammatory cells, whereas the latter are predominantly within neutrophils (or macrophages) but can also be found extracellularly scattered between inflammatory cells.[52,53] Size and shape (cocci or rods) can easily be identified using Diff Quick, and Gram staining can give additional information to classify the type of bacteria.[53] Subsequent identification and sensitivity testing will tailor appropriate antimicrobial therapy.[6,21]

Even if microorganisms were isolated from a wound, it is contraindicated to initiate systemic antimicrobial treatment if there are no clinical signs that indicate infection.[18] The former recommendation has been documented in prospective studies demonstrated that only 17% to 20% of dog bite wounds are infected,[54,55] although 84% of wounds cultured positive.[54] Most commonly cultured bacteria were *Pasteurella multocida* and *Staphylococcus intermedius* that were susceptible for cephalexin, ampicillin, and (potentiated) amoxicillin.[54] Although potentiated amoxicillin is often proposed as a first-choice antimicrobial in wound infections,[54,55] its unjustified use should be avoided because clavulanic acid is considered an emerging molecule in human medicine.[56]

DEFINITIVE TREATMENT

The objective of wound management should be either to prepare the wound to be surgically closed while minimizing the risk of infection or to control wound infection and thereby either perform delayed primary closure or promote wound healing by second intention.[5]

Host status that might impair wound healing should be addressed appropriately[57]:

- Minimize the use of systemic steroids
- Treat immunocompromising disease
- Provide adequate nutrition
- Minimize hypothermia, stress, and pain because they all increase sympathetic tone and decrease tissue perfusion

A well-vascularized wound bed provides nutrients and oxygen to sustain newly formed granulation tissue and maintains an active immunologic response to microbial invasion.[57]

Surgical Closure

Timing of wound closure depends on the location, the degree of contamination, the time from injury to treatment, as well as patient's predisposing medical conditions.[11]

Primary closure is closure of the wound before formation of granulation tissue. This method is preferred for any wound that can be converted to a clean wound.[7,21] Contaminated wounds can be converted to clean wounds by complete excision. Especially in anatomic areas where enough skin is present and no specialized tissues, such as important nerves or tendons, complete excision of the wound is the best approach.[48] Tension, potential infection, and doubtful vitality of tissues preclude primary closure.[21] Delayed primary closure allows the patient's defense system to decrease bacterial load and is typically performed after 3 to 5 days.[7,11,48] Thanks to the formation of granulation tissue, initially contaminated wounds gradually gain sufficient resistance to infection, making delayed primary closure the optimal choice in contaminated wounds.[58] In some cases, secondary healing by granulation tissue is required.[7]

Wound Dressings

If wounds cannot be treated by primary closure, a dressing should be applied to provide a physical barrier to prevent contamination and infection and to maintain a wound environment that accelerates wound healing.[1] Different types of contact layers are available with each having different applications (**Table 1**): antimicrobial effect, promotion of autolytic debridement, stimulation of granulation tissue, or stimulation of epithelialization.[21,59–61] The choice of dressing depends on the cause, size, depth, location, level of contamination, and degree of exudation of the wound.[2] A good contact layer does not adhere to the wound.[1]

Extremely dirty wounds may benefit from daily cleansing and dressing changes for the first 3 to 5 days.[4] Although the use of antimicrobial dressings is important in contaminated wounds, promotion of formation of granulation tissue is as important. Granulation tissue is resistant to infection and consequently prevents the wound from becoming infected by new contaminants from the environment.[58]

Occlusive dressings are important in healing of acute wounds. Macrophages are attracted to a moist wound environment and help to accelerate wound healing by preventing cellular dehydration and by promoting angiogenesis and autolytic debridement. Moist wound healing reduces wound pain and tenderness, fibrosis, and the risk of wound infection and also leads to a better cosmetic outcome.[57,62] Moist

Table 1 Wound dressings to promote autolytic debridement			
Agent	**Application**	**Activity**	**Contraindications**
Antimicrobial dressing (eg, honey)	12–24 h (ointment) 1–3 d (tulle)	Separation of necrosis Antimicrobial Anti-inflammatory	Large wounds, unless monitoring of hydration state, electrolytes, and protein levels, due to attraction of large amounts of fluids
Bactericidal dressing (silver dressing)	3–7 d	Antimicrobial	Necrosis
Alginate	Up to 7 d if no desiccation	Antimicrobial Promotion of granulation tissue formation	Necrosis Dry wounds, unless bandage is moistened with saline
Hydrogel	12 h–5 d	Separation of necrosis Promotion of epithelialization	Infection Moderately to highly exudative wounds Surrounding skin needs protection
Hydrocolloid	3–7 d	Necrosis	Infection Highly exudative wounds
Foam dressing	4–7 d	Separation of necrosis Large absorptive capacity Promotion of granulation tissue formation and epithelialization	Dry wounds, unless bandage is moistened with saline

Data from Refs.[59–61]

dressings are typically changed daily, and wound reassessment is planned after 3 to 4 days. If no signs of infection are present upon reexamination, delayed primary closure can be performed.[4]

Effectiveness of local antibiotic treatment is improved after gentle scrubbing of the wound with a gauze sponge moistened with saline; it not only reduces the amount of organisms present in the wound but also disrupts as well the fibrous cover, allowing the antibiotic to gain more intimate contact with bacteria.[51] Nevertheless, if acute wounds are treated correctly with regard to lavage and debridement and if the appropriate dressing in chosen, the use of local antibiotic treatment is often not necessary.[51] The use of topical antibiotics is ineffective if applied more than 3 hours after the injury.[63]

Systemic Antimicrobial Therapy

Most acute wounds do not require systemic antimicrobial treatment.[3,14] Systemic antimicrobial therapy should only be used if there is an active infection beyond the level that can be managed with local wound therapy, such as the presence of systemic signs.[18,57] If antimicrobial use is deemed appropriate, drug selection should initially be based on the most likely pathogen and their prevailing susceptibility patterns.[3,18,57] Once results of the bacteriologic culture and sensitivity are known, the antimicrobial should be switched to the smallest spectrum possible.[18]

For simple wounds, there is no evidence that the use of antimicrobials prevents the wound from becoming infected.[64] Even in dog bite wounds, debridement is more effective in reducing the infection rate than the administration of antimicrobials. High-risk dog bite wounds such as small punctures that cannot be thoroughly irrigated, on the other hand, do benefit from immediate antimicrobial therapy.[7,24] Nevertheless, deep puncture wounds should always be surgically opened, debrided, and irrigated.[24]

It has also been suggested that the administration of systemic antimicrobials in wounds treated by second-intention healing is ineffective. The rapidly developing fibrin coagulum in open wounds likely attributes to the limited access of the drug to the organisms.[51]

SUMMARY

When traumatic wounds are quickly and accurately treated, morbidity and costs can be significantly decreased. Several factors, such as time delay between injury and treatment, the degree of contamination, extension and depth of the wound, and the mechanism of injury, influence the treatment and prognosis and stress the importance of a patient-specific approach. Although all traumatic wounds are contaminated, antibiotic therapy is seldom required if correct wound management is installed.

REFERENCES

1. Percival NJ. Classification of wounds and their management. Surgery 2002;20(5): 114–7.
2. Singer AJ, Dagum AB. Current management of acute cutaneous wounds. N Engl J Med 2008;359(10):1037–46.
3. Nakamura Y, Daya M. Use of appropriate antimicrobials in wound management. Emerg Med Cin North Am 2007;25(1):159–76.
4. Nicks BA, Ayello EA, Woo K, et al. Acute wound management: revisiting the approach to assessment, irrigation, and closure considerations. Int J Emerg Med 2010;3(4):399–407.

5. Cockbill SME, Turner TD. Management of veterinary wounds. Vet Rec 1995; 136(14):362–5.
6. Dernell WS. Initial wound management. Vet Clin Small Anim 2006;36:713–38.
7. Moreira ME, Markovchick VJ. Wound management. Emerg Med Clin North Am 2007;25(3):873–99.
8. Leaper DJ, Harding KG. ABC of wound healing. Traumatic and surgical wounds. BMJ 2006;332(7540):532–5.
9. American College of Emergency Physicians. Clinical policy for the initial approach to patients presenting with penetrating extremity trauma. Ann Emerg Med 1994;23(5):1147–56.
10. Edlich RF, Rodeheaver GT, Morgan RF, et al. Principles of emergency wound management. Ann Emerg Med 1988;17(12):1284–302.
11. DeBoard RH, Rondeau DF, Kang CS, et al. Principles of basic wound evaluation and management in the emergency department. Emerg Med Clin North Am 2007;25(1):23–39.
12. Berk WA, Welch RD, Bock BF. Controversial issues in clinical management of the simple wound. Ann Emerg Med 1992;21(1):72–80.
13. Robson MC, Duke WF, Krizek TJ. Rapid bacterial screening in the treatment of civilian wounds. J Surg Res 1973;14(5):426–30.
14. Robson MC. Wound infection. A failure of wound healing caused by an imbalance of bacteria. Surg Clin North Am 1997;77(3):637–50.
15. Krizek TJ, Robson MC. Evolution of quantitative bacteriology in wound management. Am J Surg 1975;130(5):579–84.
16. Berk WA, Osbourne DD, Taylor DD. Evaluation of the 'Golden Period' for wound repair: 204 cases from a third world emergency department. Ann Emerg Med 1988;17(5):496–500.
17. Mangram AJ, Horan TC, Pearson ML, et al. Guideline for prevention of surgical site infection, 1999. Infect Control Hosp Epidemiol 1999;20(4):247–78.
18. Bowler PG, Duerden BI, Armstrong DG. Wound microbiology and associated approaches to wound management. Clin Microbiol Rev 2001;14(2):244–69.
19. Weigelt JA. Risk of wound infections in trauma patients. Am J Surg 1985;150(6): 782–4.
20. White RAS, Lane JG. Pharyngeal stick penetration injuries in the dog. J Small Anim Pract 1988;29(1):13–35.
21. Lee CK, Hansen SL. Management of acute wounds. Surg Clin North Am 2009; 89(3):659–76.
22. Gabriel A. Integrated negative pressure wound therapy system with volumetric automated fluid installation in wounds at risk for compromised healing. Int Wound J 2012;9(Suppl 1):25–31.
23. Cardany CR, Rodeheaver G, Thacker J, et al. The crush injury: a high risk wound. JACEP 1976;5(12):965–70.
24. Callaham M. Prophylactic antibiotics in common dog bite wounds: a controlled study. Ann Emerg Med 1980;9(8):410–4.
25. Alexander JW, Fischer JE, Boyajian M, et al. The influence of hair-removal methods on wound infections. Arch Surg 1983;118(3):347–52.
26. Aldridge P, O'Dwyer L. Practical emergency and critical care veterinary nursing. Chichester (United Kingdom): John Wiley & Sons; 2013.
27. Hamer ML, Robson MC, Krizek TJ, et al. Quantitative bacterial analysis of comparative wound irrigations. Ann Surg 1975;181(6):819–22.
28. Shetty R, Paul MK, Barreto E, et al. Syringe-based wound irrigating device. Indian J Plast Surg 2012;45(3):590–1.

29. Strohal R, Apelqvist J, Dissemond J, et al. EWMA document: debridement. J Wound Care 2013;22(Suppl 1):S1–52.
30. Edlich RF, Custer J, Madden J, et al. Studies in management of the contaminated wound. III. Assessment of the effectiveness of irrigation with antiseptic agents. Am J Surg 1969;118(1):21–30.
31. Custer J, Edlich RF, Prusak M, et al. Studies in the management of the contaminated wound. V. An assessment of the effectiveness of pHisoHex and Betadine surgical scrub solutions. Am J Surg 1971;121(5):572–5.
32. Stevenson TR, Thacker JG, Rodeheaver GT, et al. Cleansing the traumatic wound by high pressure syringe irrigation. JACEP 1976;5(1):17–21.
33. Wheeler CB, Rodeheaver GT, Thacker JG, et al. Side-effects of high pressure irrigation. Surg Gynecol Obstet 1976;143(5):775–8.
34. Stashak TS. Management practices that influence wound infection and healing. In: Stashak TS, Theoret C, editors. Equine wound management. 2nd edition. Ames (IA): Wiley-Blackwell; 2008. p. 85–106.
35. Chrisholm CD, Cordell WH, Rogers K, et al. Comparison of a new pressurized saline canister versus syringe irrigation for laceration cleansing in the emergency department. Ann Emerg Med 1992;21(11):1364–7.
36. Singer AJ, Hollander JE, Subramanian S, et al. Pressure dynamics of various irrigation techniques commonly used in the emergency department. Ann Emerg Med 1994;24(1):36–40.
37. Gross A, Cutright DE, Bhaskar SN. Effectiveness of pulsating water jet lavage in treatment of contaminated crushed wounds. Am J Surg 1972;124(3):373–7.
38. Brown LL, Shelton HT, Bornside GH, et al. Evaluation of wound irrigation by pulsatile jet and conventional methods. Ann Surg 1978;187(2):170–3.
39. Chatterjee JS. A critical review of irrigation techniques in acute wounds. Int Wound J 2005;2(3):258–65.
40. Campany E, Johnson RW, Whitney JD. Nurses' knowledge of wound irrigation and pressures generated during simulated wound irrigation. J Wound Ostomy Continence Nurs 2000;27(6):296–303.
41. Dire DJ, Welsh AP. A comparison of wound irrigation solutions used in the emergency department. Ann Emerg Med 1990;19(6):704–8.
42. Moscati RM, Mayrose J, Reardon RF, et al. A multicenter comparison of tap water versus sterile saline for wound irrigation. Acad Emerg Med 2007;14(5):404–9.
43. Fernandez R, Griffiths R. Water for wound cleansing. Cochrane Database Syst Rev 2012;(2):CD003861.
44. Buffa EA, Lubbe AM, Verstraete FJM, et al. The effects of wound lavage solutions on canine fibroblasts: an in vitro study. Vet Surg 1997;26(6):460–6.
45. Lammers RL, Hudson DL, Seaman ME. Prediction of traumatic wound infection with a neural network-derived decision model. Am J Emerg Med 2003;21(1):1–7.
46. Anderson D. Management of open wounds. In: Williams J, Moores A, editors. BSAVA manual of canine and feline wound management and reconstruction. 2nd edition. Gloucester (United Kingdom): British Small Animal Veterinary Association; 2009. p. 37–53.
47. Ernst AA, Gershoff L, Miller P, et al. Warmed versus room temperature saline for laceration irrigation: a randomized clinical trial. South Med J 2003;96(5):436–9.
48. Haury B, Rodeheaver G, Vensko J, et al. Debridement: an essential component of traumatic wound care. Am J Surg 1978;135(2):238–42.
49. Vowden K, Vowden P. Debridement made easy. Wounds UK 2011;7(4):1–4. Available at: http://www.wounds-uk.com/pdf/content_10133.pdf.

50. Brown A. The role of debridement in the healing process. Nurs Times 2013; 109(40):16–9.
51. Edlich RF, Madden JE, Prusak M, et al. Studies in the management of the contaminated wound. VI. The therapeutic value of gentle scrubbing in prolonging the limited period of effectiveness of antibiotics in contaminated wounds. Am J Surg 1971;121(6):668–72.
52. Thompson CA, MacNeill AL. Common infectious organisms. Vet Clin Small Anim 2017;47(1):151–64.
53. Tyler RD, Cowell RL, Meinkoth JH. Cutaneous and subcutaneous lesions. In: Cowell RL, Tyler RD, Meinkoth JH, et al, editors. Diagnostic cytology and hematology of the dog and cat. 3rd edition. St. Louis (MO): Mosby Elsevier; 2008. p. 78–111.
54. Meyers B, Schoeman JP, Goddard A, et al. The bacteriology and antimicrobial susceptibility of infected and non-infected dog bite wounds: fifty cases. Vet Microbiol 2008;127(3–4):360–8.
55. Mouro S, Vilela CL, Niza MMRE. Clinical and bacteriological assessment of dog-to-dog bite wounds. Vet Microbiol 2010;144(1–2):127–32.
56. Davies J, Davies D. Origins and evolution of antibiotic resistance. Microbiol Mol Biol Rev 2010;74(3):417–33.
57. Schultz GS, Sibbald RG, Falanga V, et al. Wound bed preparation: a systemic approach to wound management. Wound Repair Regen 2003;11(Suppl 1):1–28.
58. Edlich RF, Rogers W, Kasper G, et al. Studies in the management of the contaminated wound. I. Optimal time for closure of contaminated open wounds. II. Comparison of resistance to infection of open and closed wounds during healing. Am J Surg 1969;117(3):323–9.
59. Hosgood G. Stages of wound healing and their clinical relevance. Vet Clin North Am Small Anim Pract 2006;36(4):667–85.
60. Krahwinkel DJ, Boothe HW. Topical and systemic medications for wounds. Vet Clin North Am Small Anim Pract 2006;36(4):739–57.
61. Campbell BG. Dressings, bandages, and splints for wound management in dogs and cats. Vet Clin North Am Small Anim Pract 2006;36(4):759–91.
62. Field CK, Kerstein MD. Overview of wound healing in a moist environment. Am J Surg 1994;167(1A):2S–6S.
63. Edlich RF, Smith QT, Edgerton MT. Resistance of the surgical wound to antimicrobial prophylaxis and its mechanisms of development. Am J Surg 1973;126(5):583–91.
64. Cummings P, Del Beccaro MA. Antibiotics to prevent infection of simple wounds: a meta-analysis of randomized studies. Am J Emerg Med 1995;13(4):396–400.

Perforating Cervical, Thoracic, and Abdominal Wounds

Marije Risselada, DVM, PhD

KEYWORDS

- Body wall trauma • Body wall reconstruction • Bite wounds • Gunshot wounds

KEY POINTS

- Penetrating injuries can be associated with extensive tissue disruption and/or visceral damage.
- Bite wounds and vehicular traumas are associated with large body wall defects and less internal organ damage.
- Gunshot and impalement wounds are associated with small body wall wounds and major internal organ damage.

INTRODUCTION

Perforating wounds can be defined as any wound extending from the outside of a cavity or lumen to the inside. They can be caused by bite wounds, gunshot wounds, vehicular trauma, or other causes, such as impalement.[1–16] Most of these injuries resulting in body wall hernias are caused by bite wounds, as reported by Shaw and colleagues[7] in a retrospective series on 36 cases (26 dogs, 10 cats). Of the 26 dogs included, 14 had bite wounds, 10 had vehicular trauma, 1 was kicked by a horse, and 1 had unknown trauma.

Penetrating injuries are considered to be a serious presenting complaint regardless of the cause. A high number of surgical interventions and reconstructive procedures have been reported in the literature to be necessary.[2,14] The degree of skin damage in these cases does not give a good indication of the underlying tissue damage.[1,2,17] Radiographic evaluation of the involved body area should be included in the work-up of these patients to assess the extent of the injuries.[2,14] In most patients with penetrating injuries, severe damage to the body wall and/or internal organs is present.[1–5,18] Surgical exploration to assess the body wall and internal organs along with debridement of the underlying tissues is recommended.[4–7]

Disclosure: The author has nothing to disclose.
Department of Veterinary Clinical Sciences, College of Veterinary Medicine, Purdue University, Lynn Hall, 625 Harrison Street, West Lafayette, IN 47907, USA
E-mail address: marije_risselada@ncsu.edu

BITE WOUNDS

Bite wounds most commonly occur in small dogs. In a study of 196 bite wounds, the investigators found that small dogs ($\leq$10 kg body weight [BW]) were the most common victims (61% of dogs of the study population compared with a hospital distribution of 34%).[6] This same finding is reflected in several other studies: in a study on thoracic bite wounds, all dogs except 1 weighed less than 8 kg.[1] In a study investigating traumatic body wall herniations, bitten dogs weighed significantly less than the other included dogs (6.7 kg vs 24.3 kg BW),[7] whereas other retrospective articles reported a mean BW of bitten dogs of 5.2 kg,[2] and a median BW of 7 kg.[14]

A breed predilection for bite wounds also has been reported: The largest case series (185 dogs) found a significantly higher number of cross breeds (37%), pinschers (27%) and terriers (5%) compared with the hospital population.[6] In the article by Scheepens and colleagues,[2] a high incidence of Yorkshire terriers (27%), Jack Russell terriers (20%) and Maltese (22%) was described, whereas a different article reported a significantly higher number of Jack Russell terriers and dachshunds in the bite wound group (33.3% and 25.0% respectively).[14]

In addition, a significantly higher proportion of males than females has been reported by Shamir and colleagues,[6] and most males were intact, leading the investigators to suspect that the male predominance was most likely to be related to the influence of sex hormones. A similar finding was described in other articles.[2,14]

In the largest retrospective study[6] (185 dogs and 11 cats), the most commonly affected areas were the thorax (64 dogs; 34.5%) and the neck (57 dogs; 31%).[6] The combination of thorax and abdomen was seen in 17 out of 185 dogs (9%). This same finding is reflected in other case series, in which the most commonly area affected was the thorax and chest wall.[1,14] The thoracic cavity was involved in 6 cases (50.0%), the abdominal cavity in 2 cases (16.6%), both cavities in 2 cases (16.6%), and the trachea in 2 cases (16.6%).[14]

Radiographically, subcutaneous emphysema, effusion, rib separation, rib fractures, and pneumothorax/pneumomediastinum/pneumoperitoneum are the most commonly reported findings. Rib fractures, either single or multiple, were diagnosed in 8 patients (8 out of 12). Pneumothorax, pneumomediastinum or pneumoperitoneum, depending on the area, was present in 11 patients (11 out of 12). Effusion was noticed in 7 patients (7 out of 12). Subcutaneous emphysema was present in 11 patients (11 out of 12).[14] Two abdominal muscle disruptions were evident radiographically with organ displacement in 1 case; no intercostal muscle disruptions were suspected or seen radiographically. This finding is in contrast with previous studies that found high incidences of significant additional injuries in 75% of patients (n = 12)[19] or in 6 out of 14 patients (42%).[7]

In one study, focusing exclusively on cervical bite wounds (55 animals [38 dogs/17 cats], 56 cervical bite wounds), 31 were managed with nonsurgical wound management, 13 with only local surgery, and 10 out of 55 with a full surgical cervical exploration. Six of these 55 cases, 3 dogs and 3 cats, had airway injury (3 trachea, 3 larynx).[15] In a series of 12 bite wounds, 2 involved the cervical area: 1 required tracheal repair, whereas the other required tracheal resection and anastomosis.[14]

GUNSHOT WOUNDS

Another cause of penetrating injuries are gunshot wounds.[8,10] Patients with gunshot wounds were 0.8% of all animals examined on a yearly basis over a 5-year period in 1 hospital.[12] In human medicine, surgical exploration after penetrating abdominal gunshot wounds is considered mandatory because of the high incidence of internal organ injury.[20] This guideline has also been used in veterinary medicine.[8,21] Animals that sustained gunshot wounds had a greater amount of internal organ damage compared with bite wounds. In a retrospective human study, internal injuries were found in 67 out of 75 patients (89%) with penetrating abdominal gunshot wounds.[20] In a retrospective veterinary study, intra-abdominal injuries were found in 67% of patients, whereas gastrointestinal perforation was confirmed in 55% of patients.[19] In a more recent veterinary study, all 5 animals with evidence of peritoneal penetration had intra-abdominal injuries identified during surgery.[8]

In one article that compared bite wounds with gunshot wounds, 3 cases were included: 1 involved the abdomen only, and the 2 others involved both the thoracic and abdominal cavity. No rib fractures were found in any of the patients that were shot. No body wall disruptions were evident on radiographs and none were found surgically that needed reconstruction. However, 8 additional procedures were required because of internal organ damage.[14]

OTHER CAUSES FOR PENETRATING WOUNDS

Other causes for penetrating wounds are impalement injuries and, less commonly, vehicular trauma. Impalement injuries can be caused by objects such as arrows[22–24] or can be caused by the animal impaling itself on an object; for instance, after a fall.[13] In a case series of 3 cats with high-rise syndrome, 2 had thoracic impalement and 1 abdominal impalement. Two partial lung lobectomies were needed in 1 cat, a complete and partial lung lobectomy in the second cat with thoracic injuries, whereas a splenectomy and colon-saving procedure rather than a colonic resection and anastomosis (because of the patient's stability) were performed in the cat with abdominal wounds. Body wall defects included costochondral separation, rib trauma requiring a rib resection, and extensive soft tissue trauma necessitating a drainage technique, respectively.[13]

Soft tissue vehicular trauma injuries in dogs and cats are more commonly associated with closed body wall hernias, but these can become open if the superficial tissue and skin are damaged simultaneously. In a series of body wall hernias in 26 dogs and 10 cats reported by Shaw and colleagues,[7] 10 hernias in dogs and 3 in cats were caused by known vehicular trauma. A specific type of body wall hernia frequently seen in vehicular trauma is a prepubic hernia.[25] However, in a large cases series describing vehicular trauma in 239 dogs, fewer than 10 dogs had body wall hernias.[11]

IMAGING AND DIAGNOSTIC FINDINGS

Injuries sustained in a fight are most likely to be caused by the combination of crush, tear, and avulsion that accompanies a dog bite wound. Extensive damage to subcutaneous tissues, body wall muscles, ribs, and intercostal muscles is usually present.[1–3,9,18] Bjorling and colleagues[19] found that all animals in their study had 2 or more abnormalities and 7 animals had 4 or more abnormalities (n = 33); subcutaneous emphysema was the most common and pneumothorax the second most common reported finding.[19] In a case series intended to identify the most common causes of pneumoperitoneum in dogs and cats (39 cases), 14 were traumatic in origin: vehicular trauma (5), gunshot wounds (5), and abdominal bite wounds (2).[26]

In a case series that included both bite and gunshot wounds, subcutaneous emphysema was the most common radiographic abnormality (12 times in 16 patients).[14] This finding was more common in dogs with bite wounds than in patients that were shot. Effusion was the second most common abnormality (11 times in 16 patients). Pneumothorax and pneumoperitoneum were the third most common, and rib fractures the fourth most common abnormalities. Multiple fractures were present in 6 of these 8 patients. Subcutaneous emphysema was present in 11 out of 12 patients in the fight wound group and 1 out of 4 in the gunshot wound group. Effusion was seen in 6 out of 12 patients and 4 out of 4 patients in the respective groups. Only 2 body wall disruptions were diagnosed radiographically. Rib fractures were present in 8 cases: 1 rib was fractured in 3 cases; and 2, 3, and 4 ribs were fractured in 1 case each. Pneumothorax was radiographically evident in 7 cases, and a pneumoperitoneum in 1. Subcutaneous emphysema was evident radiographically in all but 1 of the patients. Body wall disruption was evident radiographically in 2 cases: a paracostal herniation in 1 case and a left-sided abdominal herniation in the second case.[14]

CONCURRENT INJURIES

A series investigating all concurrent injuries in cats with traumatic rib fractures (75 cases)[26] included 25 fight wounds and 13 cases with injuries from vehicular trauma. The numbers of fractures or concurrent orthopedic injuries were not associated with outcome but pleural effusion, diaphragmatic hernia, and flail chest were. Risk ratios of being more likely to die were 3.5 for diaphragmatic hernia, 3.0 for pleural effusion, and 2.1 for flail chest.[27]

In a series of 36 patients (26 dogs, 10 cats) with body wall trauma, herniated organs included intestine (13), omentum (8), bladder (3), lung (3), and liver (1), and additional surgeries that were performed were 3 small intestinal resection and anastomoses, and 1 colonic resection and anastomosis.[7] Fifteen of 26 dogs had extracavitary injuries: orthopedic (9), bite wounds needing surgical treatment (5), pulmonary contusions (3), and spinal cord injury (5), and 19 out of 26 survived. Ten cats with body wall herniation were included: 4 bite wounds, 3 vehicular trauma, and 3 of unknown causes.[7]

In a case series of 12 patients with fight and bite wounds, injury to internal organs requiring treatment (partial lung lobectomy [1], bladder repair [1]) was found only in a small number patients (2 in 12 cases; 16.6%), whereas 11 reconstructive procedures were performed.[14] No reconstructive procedures and 8 procedures for internal organ damage were required in 4 cases with gunshot wounds (**Table 1**).[14]

A similar finding was reported in case series of 11 dogs with thoracic bite wounds: only 2 incidences of visceral trauma were reported (both lung lacerations). An additional body wall defect of the abdominal wall was also reported.[1]

In a case series of 55 patients with 56 episodes of cervical bite wounds, only 14 of the 55 patients had injured vital organs requiring surgical intervention: 3 dogs and 3 cats had airway injury (3 trachea, 3 larynx). Five of these 9 patients had a primary repair performed and 1 (a cricoid laceration) was repaired with a fasciomuscular flap. Two of the 3 cats with airway injury received a temporary tracheostomy.[15]

Treatment

After stabilizing the patient, any penetrating wound into the abdominal or thoracic cavity warrants a surgical exploration. Similarly, deep cervical wounds, especially those

Table 1				
A distribution of injuries from 3 retrospective articles including multiple body areas				
	Neck	**Thorax**	**Abdomen**	**Back**
Dogs	57 out of 185[6]; 2 out of 15[14]	64 out of 185[6]; 10 out of 15[14]	44 out of 185[6]; 7 out of 15[14]	57 out of 185[6]
Cats	2 out of 11[6]	4 out of 11[6]; 1 out of 1[14]	3 out of 11[6]; 1 out of 1[14]	5 out of 11[6]

with evidence of disruption of the deeper tissue planes and/or pneumothorax and/or pneumomediastinum, should be surgically explored. Most body wall herniations (thorax and abdomen) can be repaired using autologous tissue. Use of tissue implants has been reported for treatment of large defects. Autologous tissue was used in 24 cases, and mesh in 2 cases.[7] In a case series reported by Shahar and colleagues,[1] a basket-weave pattern was used to stabilize individual ribs in dogs with thoracic bite wounds; out of the 11 dogs that were treated, 9 survived.

On surgical exploration the following body wall disruptions were found: a paracostal abdominal herniation, a diaphragmatic herniation, a caudal abdominal wall disruption, and intercostal muscle disruptions in all surgically treated thoraxes (7). Intercostal muscle disruptions ranged from 1 intercostal space to 5 intercostal spaces. Nine of these 10 herniations were repaired with autologous tissue, and in 1 thoracic wall reconstruction polypropylene mesh (Prolene, Ethicon) was used.[14]

PROGNOSIS

Hospitalization ranged from 1 to 15 days between various studies. One article reported a median number of hospitalized days of 6 for the entire group of patients (range, 3–15 days), comparable with a study of 24 cases of flail chest (dogs and cats)[28] but longer than a group of 36 patients with traumatic body wall herniation[7] or a group of 12 cases with thoracic bite wounds (range of hospitalization, 1–7 days; 2 patients treated as outpatients).[14]

Mortalities ranged from less than 1% to 39% between various reports and various causes: the mortality in a retrospective study combining different causes of perforating wounds was 11.7%,[6] whereas other studies showed mortalities of less than 1% (cervical bite wounds),[15] 11%,[8] 15%,[16] 18%,[2] 25%,[3] and 33%[19] for bitten dogs, and 19% for patients with traumatic body wall herniation[7] and 39% for gunshot wounds.[19]

Nature of the Problem

Penetrating wounds can be associated with major body wall trauma or internal organ damage. A high index of suspicion for further injuries is warranted when assessing any puncture wound.

Definition

A penetrating wound is any wound that connects a body cavity to the outside environment.

Symptom criteria:

- One or multiple wounds
- Concurrent injuries likely
- Early intervention is advisable

CLINICAL FINDINGS CERVICAL WOUNDS
Presentation and Physical Examination

Penetrating wounds in the cervical area are most often caused by bite wounds, with most of the damage incurred because of separation of tissue planes from tugging and shaking.

Several puncture wounds can be detected on physical examination, and often more become evident after widely clipping the skin in the cervical area. Bite wounds can span the entire circumference, because the damage inflicted from the bite trauma occurs from both sides. Local inflammation, edema, and emphysema are common findings (in 100% of cases reported in 2 studies).[14,15] Respiratory distress is less often seen on presentation, but its absence does not rule out injuries to the trachea or larynx.[15] If any of the major cervical vessels (jugular vein, carotid artery) are damaged, either overt bleeding or an enlarging hematoma can be present.

Diagnostic Modalities

Survey radiographs (**Fig. 1**A) can provide an indication for the presence of trauma to underlying structures, especially if separation of tracheal rings or overt trauma to the trachea (**Fig. 1**B) is present. Other modalities, such as computed tomography (CT), tracheoscopy, or esophagoscopy, can be pursued to gain more information about damage to the respiratory and/or digestive tract.[10,15]

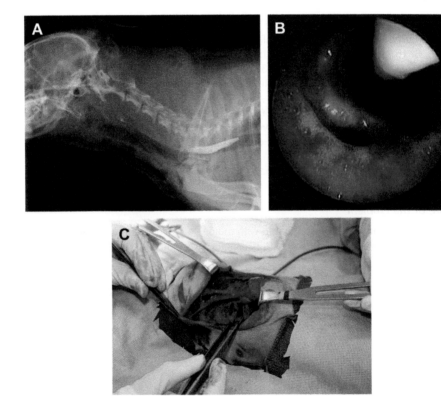

Fig. 1. A lateral cervical radiograph (*A*), tracheoscopic image (*B*), and an intraoperative image (*C*) are presented of an 8-year-old female spayed (FS) beagle that presented with cervical bite wounds. (*A*) There is subcutaneous emphysema but no discontinuity of the tracheal. (*B*) Image taken during tracheoscopy shows a ventral defect between 2 tracheal rings, spanning at least 25% of the circumference. A sterile red rubber tube can be seen passing dorsally to the endoscope, supplying O_2. (*C*) The defect in the ventral aspect of the trachea shown during midline cervical exploratory surgery. The sutures encircling the adjacent tracheal rings are preplaced before repairing the defect. A sterile endotracheal tube can be seen within the lumen of the trachea bypassing the defect. (*Courtesy of* [*A*] Southern Oaks Animal Hospital, Hope Mills, NC.)

Surgical Options

A deep cervical exploratory surgery and inspection of the trachea and esophagus is recommended if any indications of ongoing bleeding, respiratory distress, or deep tissue plane disruption are present.

Two or more separate approaches might be needed to explore all the cervical structures and wounds. The trachea and esophagus are explored through a standard ventral cervical midline position. Frequently the damage to the trachea can be repaired by reconstruction techniques using autologous tissues and suturing of the tracheal rings, similar to closure of a tracheotomy (**Fig. 1**C). Up to 25% in puppies, and 35% in adults, of the cervical trachea can be resected if a tracheal resection and anastomosis is necessary.[29] If substantial trauma to the larynx is present, necessitating surgical repair, a temporary tracheostomy can be considered during the immediate postoperative period.[15] In 56 cervical bite wounds, 6 injuries to the respiratory system requiring surgical repair were reported,[15] whereas in another study 2 incidences of tracheal trauma were reported (1 tracheal repair and 1 tracheal resection and anastomosis).[14]

Use of a feeding tube (gastrostomy tube) might be needed to rest the esophagus if extensive damage is present, or extensive repair is needed. For simple perforating wounds, a local debridement and closure might be all that is needed. At present, damage to the extent of needing an esophageal resection and anastomosis has not been described in the literature secondary to cervical bite wounds.

Care is taken not to damage the vagosympathetic trunk and recurrent laryngeal nerves on inspecting large hematomas surrounding the trachea. Both jugular veins can be ligated if needed to stop ongoing bleeding. Dogs tolerate bilateral occlusion/ligation of the carotid arteries, whereas cats do not.[30–33] Unilateral ligation of the carotid artery in dogs decreases the systolic blood pressure (BP) in the lingual artery from 104.6 to 66 mm Hg and the mean BP from 87.1 to 62 mm Hg.[31] Bilateral carotid artery ligation did not significantly decrease the BP further. Cats might not tolerate ligation of the carotid arteries as easily, because cats lack a patent internal carotid artery.[32] In one study, ligation of both carotid and vertebral arteries in cats led to cardiac arrest in 6 out of 18 animals, and respiratory changes and depression in the remaining 12.[33]

Depending on the tissue quality, primary closure or open wound management can be chosen for the more peripheral areas. If there is substantial pocketing and dead space, the different wounds can be connected to allow placement of 1 closed suction drain.

Potential Complications

Immediate complications can include respiratory distress caused by upper airway obstruction secondary to edema. Similarly, nerve damage can lead to laryngeal paralysis. Short-term complications include dehiscence of tracheal and/or esophageal repair site, wound infection, dehiscence, and tissue necrosis. Long-term complications include retained foreign material, tracheal stenosis, or esophageal stricture. Tracheal stenosis can occur after nonrepaired blunt trauma to the trachea or after repair of more extensive trauma.[29] Similarly, esophageal trauma or repair can lead to esophageal strictures.

CLINICAL FINDINGS THORACIC PENETRATING WOUNDS
Presentation and Physical Examination

Patients can present with a variety of symptoms. Most present with visible external wounds, although the lack of clearly visible perforating wounds does not rule out underlying damage and trauma. Similarly, respiratory abnormalities are present in most patients, sometimes leading to respiratory distress, although one case series reported absence of respiratory abnormalities in 1 out of 8 cases with penetrating wounds and 1 out of 13 cases with flail chest.[16]

Subcutaneous emphysema is a frequent finding in any case with puncture wounds and/or avulsion of the peripheral tissues from the underlying deeper structures. The extent of emphysema is variable from just surrounding the wounds to encompassing a large body area. An abnormal motion of the chest wall on respiration (flail chest, or pseudoflail chest) can be observed if a flail chest (a segment of ribs with 2 or more ribs, allowing the flail segment to move independently) or a pseudoflail chest (direct communication with the thoracic cavity allowing the skin to move paradoxically with respiration without a true separate flail segment of body wall) is present (**Fig. 2**). In one study, 35 dogs presented with a flail or pseudoflail chest (26 true flail, 9 pseudoflail).[3] Careful palpation may allow detection of separation of ribs and/or enlargement of the intercostal space, indicating intercostal muscle damage.[18]

The dogs with thoracic trauma have been reported as small to medium breeds: mean BW 5.2 kg, range 3.0 to 10.5 kg, 45 dogs[2]; and 6.0 kg median, range 0.4 to 32 kg, 54 dogs.[16]

Out of 65 cases, 37 cases presented within 6 hours.[16] In the same study, 27 animals had a normal respiratory pattern, 30 showed signs of dyspnea, and 8 were in

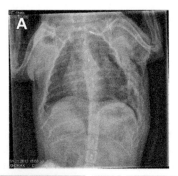

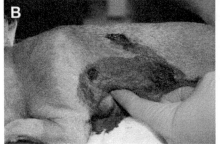
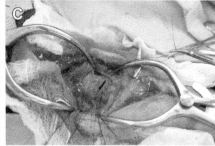

Fig. 2. A ventrodorsal projection of the thorax (*A*), a preoperative image of the anesthetized patient showing the left thoracic area (*B*), and a surgical image (*C*) of a 9-year-old FS Chihuahua. (*A*) There is subcutaneous emphysema bilaterally, pneumothorax with retraction of the left lung lobes from the chest wall, and fractures of ribs 5 to 8. (*B*) The patient in ventral recumbency is shown immediately after intubation, before clipping the chest area. Two smaller puncture wounds can be appreciated dorsally and craniolaterally, whereas a large chest wall defect can be appreciated on manual palpation. (*C*) The intraoperative image, taken after skin incision, shows the extent of underlying tissue trauma to the subcutaneous tissue, latissimus dorsi, and chest wall.

respiratory distress; 36 out of 65 had no full-thickness skin wounds, 8 had a penetrating wound (1 out of 8 normal respiratory pattern, 2 in respiratory distress), and 13 were diagnosed with a flail chest (1 out of 13 normal respiratory pattern, 2 in respiratory distress). Radiographic lesions included pulmonary contusions in 26 patients (23 dogs, 3 cats), rib fractures in 23 patients (21 dogs, 2 cats), pneumothorax in 17 (13 dogs, 4 cats), and pleural effusion in 8 patients (7 dogs, 1 cat). Treatment included conservative management (37) and exploratory surgery (10 local explore, 18 thoracotomy). Ten of the 65 patients did not survive, of which 5 were euthanized before treatment.[16]

Diagnostic Modalities

Radiographs remain the mainstay as the initial imaging modality to assess the extent of injury. Thoracic-focused assessment with sonography for trauma can be used to check for pleural effusion, but any presence of subcutaneous air makes ultrasonographic assessment difficult. One study concluded that penetrating injury and/or more than 3 radiographic lesions was an indication for thoracotomy.[16] Absence of these features is an indication for surgical exploration that might need to be converted to thoracotomy. CT scans have been shown to be more sensitive in detecting rib fractures than radiographs, and are now commonly performed during the work-up for trauma in human patients[34] as well as in veterinary patients.

The most common findings are subcutaneous emphysema, pneumothorax, pulmonary contusion, and rib fractures.[18] Rib fractures, either single or multiple, were diagnosed in 8 patients (8 out of 12). Pneumothorax, pneumomediastinum, or pneumoperitoneum, depending on the area, was present in 11 patients (11 out of 12). Effusion was noticed in 7 patients (7 out of 12). Subcutaneous emphysema was present in 11 patients (11 out of 12). Two abdominal muscle disruptions were evident radiographically with organ displacement in 1 case, and no intercostal muscle disruptions were suspected or seen radiographically.[14]

In the fight wound group, body wall disruption was evident surgically in 8 patients. Eleven separate reconstructive procedures were performed in the 8 patients with body wall disruptions. In 1 case, polypropylene mesh was used for thoracic wall reconstruction. All other reconstructions were performed using autogenous tissue only. Tracheal repair was required in 1 case and tracheal resection and anastomosis in another. Therefore, a total of 13 separate reconstructive procedures were performed in 10 patients. Additional procedures were partial lung lobectomy (1) and bladder repair (1) (**Table 2**). In 1 dog with both a ruptured bladder and a flail chest, the flail chest was managed conservatively without a splint after an exploratory celiotomy and bladder repair were performed.

Surgical Options

Surgical options include, but are not limited to, surgical exploration, stabilization, external stabilization without exploration, and chest wall reconstruction techniques (flaps, omental advancement, synthetic materials, [porcine] small intestinal submucosa [SIS], basket weave pattern).[1,17,35,36]

While stabilizing the patient before surgery, or if surgery is not an option for the owner, the flail chest can be temporarily treated by placing the patient flail side down, or with a bandage that restricts the motion of the segment but does not affect respiratory function. An external stabilizing method using circumcostal sutures tied to a rigid device placed on the skin (plastic; a synthetic cast or a frame) has been described.[36]

Table 2
Concurrent internal injuries necessitating surgical repair listed per cause and body area

	Bite	Gunshot	Impalement
Thorax	Lung: 2 out of 11[1]; 13 out of 45[2]; 1 out of 12[14] Abdominal wall: 1 out of 11[1] Diaphragmatic hernia 3 out of 45[2]	Lung: 2 out of 4[14]	Lung: 2 out of 2[13]
Abdomen	Bladder repair: 1 out of 12[14]	Small intestine: 3 out of 4[14] Bladder: 1 out of 4[14]	Spleen: 1 out of 1[13]
Neck	Injuries to vital structures: 14 out of 55[15] Airway: 6 out of 55[15] Trachea: 2 out of 2[14]		

The simplest method of stabilization and reconstructing chest wall defects is to place circumcostal sutures around 2 ribs spanning a defect or in a basket-weave pattern to stabilize mobile segments, as described by Shahar and colleagues.[1] This technique uses autologous tissue (adjacent ribs) to stabilize mobile rib segments, and allows a quick reconstruction of the chest wall, while avoiding placing a foreign body (such as a mesh) in a contaminated area.

For larger defects, an implant, such as a surgical mesh, or SIS can be used to reconstruct the chest wall. An omental flap can be harvested from the abdomen and tunneled through the diaphragm or subcutaneously for additional support. In cases with severe local muscle and skin loss, an axial pattern flap can be rotated into the defect for additional coverage.

In human medicine, a flail chest is defined as unilateral fractures of 4 or more ribs, with each rib fractured in 2 or more locations, whereas a clinical flail chest is diagnosed if the segment is large enough to allow paradoxic motion of the chest wall with respiration.[34] Indications to treat chest wall injuries surgically in people are the presence of flail chest, in order to reduce pain, if a chest wall defect/deformity is present, if a thoracotomy is needed for other indications such as pulmonary or cardiac trauma, and the presence of open fractures.[34] Non–surgically-treated human patients in several articles needed more ventilator support and had less chest wall stability compared with surgically treated patients.[34]

Operative techniques in human surgery for chest wall defects include muscle-sparing techniques.[34] Early open reduction internal fixation (ORIF) reduces the extent of thoracic wall dissection needed. Fixation options that are used frequently for ORIF are plates and nails. Metal plates are the most common and standard choice, whereas absorbable plates made from absorbable polymer, fixed in place with absorbable suture, are used as well. Absorbable plates can minimize stress shielding and do not require a second surgery. Intramedullary fixation has been used but is technically demanding. The use of Judet struts (bendable metal plates that grip the ribs at both sites, eliminating the need for screws) and U plates using locking screws has been described as well.

Nolff and colleagues[35] recently described the use of negative pressure wound therapy (NPWT) with instillation plus mesh for body wall reconstruction in a dachshund. (See Bryden J. Stanley's article, "Negative Pressure Wound Therapy," in this issue, for a more detailed discussion.)

Potential complications include pulmonary contusions, arrhythmogenic cardiac trauma, pyothorax, and sequestrum formation of loose rib fragments. Patients with pulmonary contusions might require mechanical ventilation in severe cases.[37] Cardiac arrhythmias caused by trauma can occur up to 2 days after a traumatic event.[38]

Pyothorax can occur after surgical exploratory thoracotomy, or can occur in cases without a full exploratory surgery.

CLINICAL FINDINGS: ABDOMINAL PENETRATING WOUNDS
Physical Examination

Patients can present with a variety of symptoms. Most present with visible external wounds (**Fig. 3**), although the lack of clearly visible perforating wounds does not rule out underlying damage and trauma. A high index of suspicion for perforating abdominal wounds/body wall disruption is needed for all small patients with wounds over the midabdominal to ventral abdominal area. Similarly, the presence/absence of a prepubic hernia or prepubic tendon avulsion needs to be investigated in patients with pelvic trauma that includes pubic fractures and bruising along the ventral aspect of the abdomen. The presenting signs can be nonspecific, and the final diagnosis might not be made until exploratory surgery is performed.[25]

Other symptoms or presenting complaints can be secondary to internal organ injury, such as uroabdomen, septic abdomen, bile peritonitis, or hemoabdomen.

Diagnostic modalities include survey radiographs, abdominal focused assessment with sonography for trauma, a full abdominal ultrasonographic assessment, or a trauma CT.

Loss of the ventral abdominal stripe indicates a ventral abdominal hernia, and is evidence of intra-abdominal organs in the subcutaneous space. Presence of loss of the ventral abdominal stripe with displacement of fragments of bone of the pubic rim indicates a prepubic hernia.[25] Pneumoperitoneum indicates a perforating wound or rupture of a hollow viscus, but its absence does not preclude a perforating wound, especially in gunshot wounds.[10]

Rib fractures, either single or multiple, were diagnosed in 8 patients (8 out of 12). Pneumothorax, pneumomediastinum, or pneumoperitoneum, depending on the area, was present in 11 patients (11 out of 12). Effusion was noted in 7 patients (7 out of 12). Subcutaneous emphysema was present in 11 patients (11 out of 12). Two abdominal muscle disruptions were evident radiographically, with organ displacement in 1 case.[14]

Surgical Options

Abdominal wall defects can include just the abdominal wall or can be a combination of a diaphragmatic and paracostal abdominal wall defect. A prepubic tendon avulsion is

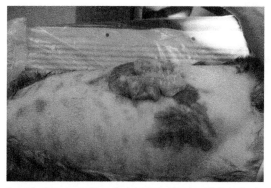

Fig. 3. A domestic short hair presenting after an impalement injury is shown. The omentum can be seen protruding from a full-thickness abdominal wall defect.

a specific type of abdominal wall defect because it often requires drilling of bone tunnels for reattachment rather than relying on soft tissue reconstructive techniques only.[25]

Timing of surgical repair depends on the overall stability of the patient (in order to undergo anesthesia), the size of the defect (and the likelihood of organs getting incarcerated and/or strangulated in the hernia), and concurrent injuries that necessitate surgical exploration (such as trauma to the abdominal organs and perforating abdominal wounds). In cases with a large abdominal defect with or without organ damage or communicating wounds, repair can be delayed for several days if necessary to allow stabilization.[25] Although tissue might retract further over the course of several days, the holding strength of the remaining tissue might be increased after the initial inflammatory phase has subsided.

A standard midline exploration is the preferred method that allows access to and assessment of all intra-abdominal structures. Ideally the hernia is reconstructed and closed before exploring the superficial, external portion of the bite wounds. In most cases, autologous tissues can be used for herniorrhaphy. Nolff and colleagues[39] recently described the use of NPWT with instillation plus mesh for body wall reconstruction in a dachshund.

Care must be taken to take large enough bites if a soft tissue reconstruction is performed for a prepubic hernia. The preferred method for prepubic tendon avulsion or prepubic hernia repair is to drill holes through the pubic bone in order to reattach the fascia to the pelvis.[25] Ideally, nonabsorbable sutures are used for the repair in a tension-relieving suture pattern. A nonabsorbable mesh can be used to augment the repair or to replace the caudal portion of the body wall if retraction has occurred and reattachment would place too much tension on the repair.

Potential Complications

Most of the risks for postoperative complications depend on the potential for ongoing wound infection and tissue necrosis. Other risks can be secondary to specific surgeries needed to address intra-abdominal visceral trauma.

Loss of domain can become an issue in chronic wounds or if a large defect is repaired with autologous tissues only. Options to prevent loss of domain are to use synthetic mesh to avoid limiting or decreasing the intra-abdominal space, or in rare cases to perform a splenectomy in order to make more room available in the abdominal cavity.

Closed suction drains can be used to monitor postoperative abdominal effusion after abdominal closure.[40,41]

SUMMARY

Penetrating injuries can be associated with extensive tissue disruption (bite wounds) and/or visceral damage (bite wounds, gunshot wounds, impalement injuries). Early exploration and appropriate wound management are indicated.

REFERENCES

1. Shahar R, Shamir M, Johnston DE. A technique for management of bite wounds of the thoracic wall in small dogs. Vet Surg 1997;26:45–50.
2. Scheepens ETF, Peeters ME, L'eplattenier HF, et al. Thoracic bite trauma in dogs: a comparison of clinical and radiological parameters with surgical results. J Small Anim Pract 2006;47:721–6.

3. Neal TM, Key JC. Principles of treatment of dog bite wounds. J Am Anim Hosp Assoc 1976;12:657–60.
4. Cowell AK, Penwick RC. Dog bite wounds: a study of 93 cases. Comp Contin Educ Pract Vet 1989;11:313–20.
5. Holt DE, Griffin G. Bite wounds in dogs and cats. Vet Clin North Am Small Anim Pract 2000;30:669–79.
6. Shamir MH, Leisner S, Klement E, et al. Dog bite wounds in dogs and cats: a retrospective study of 196 cases. J Vet Med A Physiol Pathol Clin Med 2002; 49:107–12.
7. Shaw SP, Rozanski EA, Rush JE. Traumatic body wall herniation in 36 dogs and cats. J Am Anim Hosp Assoc 2003;39:35–46.
8. Fullington RJ, Otto CM. Characteristics and management of gunshot wounds in dogs and cats: 84 cases (1986-1995). J Am Vet Med Assoc 1997;210:658–62.
9. Davidson EB. Managing bite wounds in dogs and cats. Comp Contin Educ Pract Vet 1998;20:811–20.
10. Pavletic MM, Trout NJ. Bullet, bite, and burn wounds in dogs and cats. Vet Clin Small Anim 2006;36:873–93.
11. Streeter EM, Rozanski EA, de Laforcade-Buress A, et al. Evaluation of vehicular trauma in dogs: 239 cases (January-December 2001). J Am Vet Med Assoc 2009;235:405–8.
12. Olsen LE, Streeter EM, DeCook RR. Review of gunshot injuries in cats and dogs and utility of a triage scoring system to predict short-term outcome: 37 cases (2003-2008). J Am Vet Med Assoc 2014;245(8):923–9.
13. Pratschke KM, Kirby BM. High rise syndrome with impalement in three cats. J Small Anim Pract 2002;43:261–4.
14. Risselada M, de Rooster H, Taeymans O, et al. Penetrating injuries in dogs and cats. A study of 16 cases. Vet Comp Orthop Traumatol 2008;21:434–9.
15. Jordan CJ, Halfacree ZJ, Tivers MS. Airway injury associated with cervical bite wounds in dogs and cats: 56 cases. Vet Comp Orthop Traumatol 2013;26:89–93.
16. Cabon Q, Deroy C, Ferrand F-X, et al. Thoracic bite trauma in dogs and cats: a retrospective study of 65 cases. Vet Comp Orthop Traumatol 2015;28:448–54.
17. Orton EC. Thoracic wall. In: Slatter D, editor. Textbook of small animal surgery, vol. 1, 3rd edition. Philadelphia: WB Saunders; 2003. p. 373–86.
18. McKiernan BC, Adams WM, Hulse DC. Thoracic bite wounds and associated internal injuries in 11 dogs and 1 cat. J Am Vet Med Assoc 1994;184:959–64.
19. Bjorling DE, Crowe DT Jr, Kolata RJ, et al. Penetrating abdominal wounds in dogs and cats. J Am Anim Hosp Assoc 1982;18:742–8.
20. McCarthy MC, Lowdermilk GA, Canal DF, et al. Prediction of injury caused by penetrating wounds to the abdomen, flank, and back. Arch Surg 1991;126: 962–5.
21. Kirby BM. Peritoneum and peritoneal cavity. In: Slatter D, editor. Textbook of small animal surgery, vol. 1, 3rd edition. Philadelphia: WB Saunders; 2003. p. 414–45.
22. Popish JR. Thoracic and abdominal arrow wound in the cat. J Am Vet Med Assoc 1958;15:512–3.
23. Mills MT. An unsuspected arrow wound in a dog. Vet Med Small Anim Clin 1977; 72:553.
24. Jeffrey KL, Bradley R. Thoracic and abdominal wound in a cat shot with an arrow. Vet Med Small Anim Clin 1981;76:353–4.
25. Beittenmiller MR, Mann FA, Constaninescu GM, et al. Clinical anatomy and surgical repair of prepubic hernia in dogs and cats. J Am Anim Hosp Assoc 2009;45: 284–90.

26. Saunders WB, Tobias KM. Pneumoperitoneum in dogs and cats: 39 cases (1983-2002). J Am Vet Med Assoc 2003;223:462–8.

27. Kraje BJ, Kraje AC, Rohrbach BW, et al. Intrathoracic and concurrent orthopedic injury associated with traumatic rib fracture in cats: 75 cases (1980-1998). J Am Vet Med Assoc 2000;216:51–4.

28. Olsen D, Renberg W, Perrett J, et al. Clinical management of flail chest in dogs and cats: a retrospective study of 24 cases (1989-1999). J Am Anim Hosp Assoc 2002;38:315–20.

29. Nelson AW. Diseases of the trachea and bronchi. In: Slatter D, editor. Textbook of small animal surgery. 3rd edition. Philadelphia: WB Saunders; 2002. p. 858–79.

30. Badylak S, Kokini K, Tullius B, et al. Strength over time of a resorbable bioscaffold for body wall repair in a dog model. J Surg Res 2001;99:282–7.

31. Holmberg DL, Pettifer GR. The effect of carotid artery occlusion on lingual arterial blood pressure in dogs. Can Vet J 1997;38(10):629–31.

32. Gillilan LA. Extra- and intra-cranial blood supply to brains of dog and cat. Am J Anat 1976;146(3):237–53.

33. Holmes RL, Wolstencroft JH. Accessory sources of blood supply to the brain of the cat. J Physiol 1959;148:93–107.

34. Lafferty PM, Anavian J, Will RE, et al. Operative treatment of chest wall injuries: indications, technique, and outcome. J Bone Joint Surg Am 2011;93:97–110.

35. Nolff MC, Pieper K, Meyer-Lindenberg A. Treatment of a perforating thoracic bite wound in a dog with negative pressure wound therapy. J Am Vet Med Assoc 2016;249:794–800.

36. Orton EC. Disorders of the thoracic wall. In: Orton EC, editor. Small animal thoracic surgery. Malvern (PA): Williams & Wilkins; 1995. p. 73–83.

37. Campbell VL, King LG. Pulmonary function, ventilator management, and outcome of dogs with thoracic trauma and pulmonary contusions: 10 cases (1994-1998). J Am Vet Med Assoc 2000;217(10):1505–9.

38. Macintire DK, Snider TG 3rd. Cardiac arrhythmias associated with multiple trauma in dogs. J Am Vet Med Assoc 1984;184:541–5.

39. Nolff MC, Layer A, Meyer-Lindenberg A. Negative pressure wound therapy with instillation for body wall reconstruction using an artificial mesh in a dachshund. Aust Vet J 2015;93:367–72.

40. Mueller MG, Ludwig LL, Barton LJ. Use of closed-suction drains to treat generalized peritonitis in dogs and cats: 40 cases (1997-1999). J Am Vet Med Assoc 2001;219:789–94.

41. Szabo SD, Jermyn K, Neel J, et al. Evaluation of postceliotomy peritoneal drain fluid volume, cytology, and blood-to-peritoneal fluid lactate and glucose differences in normal dogs. Vet Surg 2011;40(4):444–9.

Systemic and Local Management of Burn Wounds

Alessio Vigani, DVM, PhD*, Christine A. Culler, DVM, MS

KEYWORDS

- Burn injury • Hypermetabolic syndrome • Burn care • Fluid resuscitation
- Smoke inhalation • Burn shock

KEY POINTS

- Management of a patient with a severe burn injury is a long-term process addressing the local burn wound care and immediate and progressive systemic consequences of the injury.
- Critical aspects of emergency and intensive care management of severe burns include fluid resuscitation, cardiovascular stabilization, respiratory support, pain control, and local management of burn wounds.
- Respiratory injury should be highly suspected in burn patients, particularly with severe burns.
- Patients with more than 15% of total body surface area nonsuperficial burns are at risk of developing burn shock and require attentive fluid therapy and gastric ulcer prophylaxis.
- Profound and persistent metabolic changes are seen in patients with severe burns.

INTRODUCTION

A severe burn is any burn injury that is complicated by major trauma or inhalation injury, chemical burn, high-voltage electrical burn, and in general any nonsuperficial burn encompassing more than 20% of the total body surface area (TBSA).[1] Management of a patient with a severe burn injury is a long-term process that addresses the local burn wound care as well as the immediate and progressive systemic consequences of the injury. Critical aspects of emergency and intensive care management of severe burns include fluid resuscitation, cardiovascular stabilization, respiratory support, pain control, and local management of burn wounds.[2,3]

The authors have nothing to disclose.
Department of Clinical Sciences, North Carolina State University, College of Veterinary Medicine, 1052 William Moore Drive, Raleigh, NC 27607, USA
* Corresponding author.
E-mail address: avigani@ncsu.edu

Vet Clin Small Anim 47 (2017) 1149–1163
http://dx.doi.org/10.1016/j.cvsm.2017.06.003
0195-5616/17/© 2017 Elsevier Inc. All rights reserved.

Three major risk factors for mortality in humans with severe burns are:

- Advanced age,
- Nonsuperficial burns covering more than 40% of the TBSA, and
- Inhalation injury.

Despite major advances in the management of patients with severe burns—including patient-targeted resuscitation, management of inhalation injuries, specific nutritional support, enhanced wound therapy, and infection control—the consequences of severe burns often result in complex metabolic changes that may involve every organ system.

Consensus guidelines and clinical evidence regarding the specific management of small animal burn patients are lacking. This article aims to review updated therapeutic consideration for the systemic and local management of severe burns that are proven effective to optimize patient care and outcomes in human burn patients and likely are effective in small animal patients.

CLASSIFICATION OF BURN WOUNDS

Burns are classified by their depth of injury and by the extent of TBSA affected. This information can be helpful to determine the severity of the burn, anticipate potential sequelae, guide treatment planning, and establish expectations with owners regarding cost, duration of treatment, and extent of cosmetic recovery.

Depth of Burn Wound

Classifying wounds by degree (ie, first, second, third degree) has been replaced by the currently favored method of classification based on depth. **Table 1** describes the appearance of the various types of burns and examples of each are shown in **Fig. 1**. Superficial burns involve only the epidermis and result in no systemic effects, with relatively rapid and cosmetic healing.[4] These burns are painful and erythematous. Superficial partial thickness burns include all of the epidermis and a superficial portion of the dermis. Deep partial thickness burns comprise the entirety of the epidermis and dermis. Full-thickness burns encompass the epidermis, all of the dermis, and extend into the hypodermis.

Burns are often heterogenous, including both superficial and deep lesions. Additionally, burn wounds may evolve over a number of days, necessitating daily reclassification of the burn until the injury has declared itself fully.[4,5] This is particularly true in areas of thin skin, such as the ears and medial thighs; wounds in these areas are rarely merely superficial.[5]

Treatment strategies vary somewhat for each type of wound, as described in **Table 1**. Intuitively, healing for deeper wounds will take longer and require more aggressive and complex care than superficial wounds (see **Table 1**).

Extent of Burn Wounds

The extent of burn size is crucial to guide treatment and help with client discussion about cost and expectations. Unfortunately, no accurate method currently exists in veterinary medicine to facilitate estimation of TBSA affected. Given the diversity of conformations within veterinary patients, translation of the human estimates onto our patients will inevitably be inaccurate. For example, the short limbs of a dachshund are unlikely to represent the same relative percent of TBSA as a Labrador. Until another method of estimation is determined, however, using human guidelines as a rough estimate may be helpful, remembering to adjust interpretation based on variations in breeds.

Table 1
Classification of burn wounds based on depth of tissue injury

Classification	Depth	Appearance	Pain	Healing
Superficial	Epidermis	• Dry, red • Blanch • No blisters	• Painful	• 3–6 d • Re-epithelialization • Minimal scarring
Superficial partial-thickness	Epidermis Superficial dermis	• Erythematous • Moist, weeping • Blanch • Blisters • Eschar	• Painful with air and temperature	• 1–3 wk • Re-epithelialization • Minimal to no scarring
Deep partial-thickness	Epidermis Deep dermis	• Variable, mottled color • Waxy or wet • No blanching • Blisters • Eschar	• Reduced sensation • Pain with pressure only	• 2–3+ weeks • Scarring variable • Surgical intervention reduces scarring
Full thickness	Epidermis Dermis Hypodermis	• Bloodless • Varied: waxy white, leathery, gray to black • Dry, inelastic • No blanching • No blisters • Eschar • Easily plucked hair	• Pain with deep pressure only • May not be painful	• Requires surgery • Severe scarring with contracture

The full extent of TBSA that is affected may not be apparent until the wound has fully declared itself, which may take 3 days or more.[4,5] It is important to know that the percent TBSA affected is often deceptively less at presentation, because wounds evolve with time and eschar separation.

Rule of nines
The "rule of nines" can be used to approximate the extent of TBSA that is affected by a burn in adults. This approach assigns a percentage of TBSA to each of the following: head and neck, anterior thorax, posterior thorax, anterior abdomen, posterior abdomen, each forelimb, anterior aspect of each rear limb, and the posterior aspect of each rear limb (**Table 2**).[6,7]

Lund–Browder chart
In adults and children, the Lund–Browder chart is the most accurate way of estimating TBSA. Growth affects the relationship between areas of the body, with children having proportionally smaller legs and larger heads than adults.[4,8] Images with full details for this approach may be readily found elsewhere.

Classification of burn based on total body surface area
Burns affecting less than 20% of the TBSA are classified as a local burn, whereas those affecting more than 20% to 30% are classified as a severe burn injury (**Table 3**).

A 2008 study in humans found a significant association ($P<.001$) between nonsurvival and percent of total TBSA affected, as well as percent of full-thickness burns.[9]

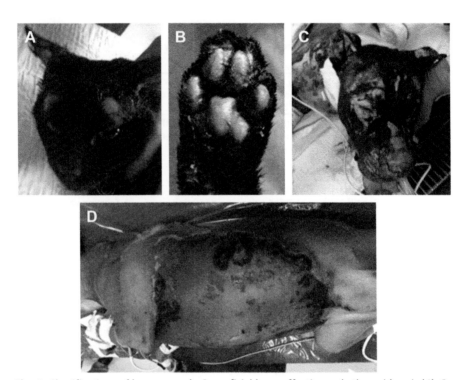

Fig. 1. Classifications of burn wounds. Superficial burn affecting only the epidermis (*A*). Superficial partial thickness burn, affecting the epidermis and the superficial part of the dermis (*B*). Deep partial thickness burn, affecting the epidermis and entirety of the dermis (*C*). Full-thickness burn, extending into the hypodermis (*D*).

In humans, patients with severe burn injury are often cared for in the intensive care unit of a burn center because they are at risk for systemic inflammatory response and organ dysfunction.[10] A retrospective review found burn wounds covering more than 40% of the TBSA to be a risk factor for death.[2] The Baux score (age + TBSA) has been shown in people to predict mortality and a recent retrospective study determined the point of futility (a score of 160), at which the predicted mortality was 100%.[11] This score may assist with the instigation of palliative care, rather than pursuit of burn treatment. No such score yet exists for veterinary medicine.

Table 2
Rule of nines for estimation of total body surface area in humans affected by a burn

Area	Percentage (%)	Total Percent
Head and neck	9	9
Each arm	9	18
Each leg	18	36
Anterior trunk	18	18
Posterior trunk	18	18
Genitalia	1	1

Table 3	
Classification of burn based on total body surface area affected by a burn	
Percent Body Surface Area Affected	**Classification of Burn**
<20	Local burn
>20-30	Severe burn injury

Zones of Burn Wound

Three dynamic zones may make up a wound: zone of coagulation and necrosis, zone of stasis, and zone of hyperemia.[10] These zones are determined by the degree of tissue perfusion and the relationship to the margin of the wound (**Table 4**).

TRIAGE AND EMERGENCY STABILIZATION

Emergency care of the burn patient follows the principles of the Advanced Trauma Life Support guidelines focusing on stabilizing the airway, breathing, and circulation (ABCs). The primary survey includes identification of respiratory distress and possible smoke inhalation injury, evaluating cardiovascular status and evidence of shock, identification of concurrent injuries, and determining the severity (superficial, partial or full thickness) and extent (TBSA) of the burn.[12]

Patient stabilization begins at admission and continues in the intensive care unit. Critical steps in stabilizing the severe burn patient are represented by airway management and respiratory support if necessary, fluid resuscitation, cardiovascular stabilization, pain control, and immediate burn care.

Airway Management and Respiratory Support

It is critical to provide supplemental oxygen and maintain the airway in patients with major burns. The risk of inhalation injury increases with the extent of the burn and the inhalation of hot gases generally induces primary damage to the upper airway with secondary edema that can occur rapidly.[13] Often patients who manifest signs of smoke inhalation are at high risk of complete airway obstruction and should be monitored very closely. Patients with severe burns often require tracheal intubation. An initial assessment may reveal no evidence of injury, but laryngeal edema can develop suddenly and unexpectedly.[14]

Early clinical signs suggestive of inhalation injury are:

- Respiratory distress,
- Persistent cough and stridor,
- Depressed mental status,
- Dark colored sputum in the mouth, and
- Blistering or edema of the oropharynx.

Table 4			
Zones of a burn wound and perfusion and healing characteristics for each			
Zone	**Location**	**Tissue Perfusion**	**Tissue Recovery**
Coagulation and necrosis	Wound center	None	Irreversible damage
Stasis	Surrounding central zone of coagulation	Decreased	May recover with aggressive management
Hyperemia	Wound periphery	Good	Likely

It is indicated to obtain thoracic radiographs and arterial blood gas analysis in all patients with respiratory signs after burn injury. Monitoring of end-tidal CO_2 ($EtCO_2$) with capnography also can provide useful real-time information about respiratory status, adequacy of resuscitation, and potential cyanide toxicity. In dogs, the use of nasal cannulas has been shown to be reliable at assessing $EtCO_2$ in nonintubated patients.

Burn patients are often exposed to carbon monoxide and cyanide, and potential poisoning should be suspected in any patient with signs of inhalation injury.[13] Standard pulse oximetry is not reliable with significant carbon monoxide toxicity. Carboxyhemoglobin has a light wavelength absorption very similar to oxyhemoglobin and standard pulse oximetry will display an SpO_2 approximating 99% even in presence of severe hypoxemia. Standard arterial blood gas also cannot establish or exclude carbon monoxide or cyanide intoxication.

Carbon monoxide toxicity requires immediate oxygen supplementation and possibly hyperbaric oxygen therapy. Treatment with high-flow oxygen alone effectively removes carbon monoxide and the possible advantages of hyperbaric oxygen remain controversial.[14]

The possibility of cyanide toxicity should also be suspected in presence of signs of inhalation injury. Serial serum lactate measurements and $EtCO_2$ monitoring during resuscitation may provide useful information at determining the likelihood of cyanide poisoning. Cyanide toxicity disrupts cellular active phosphorylation, forcing the organism to anaerobic metabolism. This change results in persistent and severe lactic acidosis despite hemodynamic stabilization and a secondary compensatory decrease in $EtCO_2$. Cyanide poisoning requires antidotal therapy. Treatment for cyanide toxicity should be initiated in burn patients with respiratory signs, unexplained severe lactic acidosis, and hypocapnia. The treatment of choice is high-dose hydroxocobalamin given as a single intravenous infusion at 70 mg/kg; a second dose of 35 mg/kg may be repeated depending on the clinical response of the patient.[15]

Patients with severe burns are at risk of developing acute respiratory distress syndrome. Should mechanical ventilation be required, lung protective strategies with use of low tidal volume ventilation and permissive hypercapnia are recommended. Despite advances in respiratory support, inhalation injury remains a leading cause of mortality in burn victims.[14] Many additional interventions are currently being investigated for the optimization of care for these patients. Bronchodilators may be considered when bronchospasm is suspected. The use of corticosteroids has been associated with an increased risk of bacterial infection and is contraindicated.[16] A novel approach is the use of aerosolized heparin and N-acetylcysteine to facilitate the removal of bronchial casts and is currently under scrutiny.[17,18]

Fluid Resuscitation

Burn shock often occurs during the first 24 to 48 hours after severe burns. It is characterized by increased capillary permeability and myocardial depression leading to large fluid shifts and secondary vascular collapse owing to depletion of intravascular volume.[19] Patient with greater than 15% TBSA nonsuperficial burns are at high risk of developing burn shock.[12] Volume depletion is the most common cause of hemodynamic instability and decreased urine output in the burn patient. Clinical signs of volume status, such as heart rate, blood pressure, pulse pressure, peripheral pulse quality, capillary refill time, and intact skin temperature of extremities are closely monitored for the first 24 hours. An indwelling catheter is useful to monitor urine output, which should be maintained at 0.5 mL/kg or greater during ongoing resuscitation. A low mixed venous oxygen saturation and an increased serum lactate also suggest poor tissue perfusion and are useful tools to monitor patient response to stabilization.

Immediate fluid resuscitation is targeted to rapidly reconstitute intravascular volume and correct hypotension if present. Ongoing fluid resuscitation is then necessary during the first 24 to 48 hours to maintain end-organ perfusion.[20] Delayed and inadequate fluid resuscitation have been shown to be associated with increased mortality.[21]

Fluid requirements during the initial 24 hours are conventionally calculated using formulas based on the TBSA involved by nonsuperficial burns. In humans, the Parkland–Baxter and the Brooke formulas are often used. These formulas estimate fluid requirements during the initial 24 hours of 4 and 2 mL/kg, respectively, for each percent of TBSA burned.[22] One-half of the calculated fluid need is given in the first 8 hours, and the remaining amount is given over the subsequent 16 hours. According to 1 retrospective review, use of the modified Brooke formula may reduce the total volume used in fluid resuscitation without causing harm.[23]

Balanced isotonic type fluids are recommended for intravenous fluid resuscitation to reduce the incidence of hyperchloremic acidosis that may occur with administration of large volumes of isotonic saline. The use of hypertonic saline or colloids for resuscitation is controversial and did not improve survival when compared with crystalloids.[24,25] The rate of infusion for intravenous resuscitation fluids should be as constant as possible; rapid decreases or increases in infusion rates can lead to vascular collapse and an increase in edema respectively.

Although adequate fluid resuscitation is crucial, care should be taken not to overresuscitate. Severely burned patients require a large amount of fluid during resuscitation that can contribute to the development of volume overload, intraabdominal hypertension, and compartment syndrome.[26,27] Overresuscitation is associated with severe consequences, including worsening of edema, acute respiratory distress syndrome, multiorgan failure, and abdominal or extremity compartment syndromes.[28,29] Patients at risk for extremity compartment syndrome are closely monitored for peripheral neurologic function and perfusion to determine immediate need for escharotomy, discussed in more detail elsewhere in this article. This risk reinforces the importance of using formulas only as initial approximation of fluid resuscitation needs and then carefully following a patient-oriented approach, continually adjusting resuscitation efforts according to the physiologic response.[27]

Analgesia, Sedation, and Anxiolysis

Pain management represents a critical component of the stabilization of burn patients. Human burn patients typically report pain as being severe or excruciating. Burn pain shows substantial variations over the course of hospitalization, with often unpredictable worsening despite aggressive analgesia (**Table 5**).[30] Background burn pain can be unbearable, especially in the presence of extensive partial thickness burns. They are associated with marked hyperalgesia secondary to injury and inflammation of sensory receptors in the dermis. Full-thickness burns are counterintuitively associated

Table 5
Types of pain associated with burn wounds and the nature of each

Type of Pain	Character of Pain	Circumstances
Background	• Dull • Constant	• Related to extent and degree of burn
Procedural	• Sharp • Lasts minutes to hours	• Medical or nursing care interventions • May be anticipatory
Breakthrough	• Sharp, severe	• Triggered by movement

with decreased tissue sensitivity; however, the area surrounding a full-thickness burn is extremely hypersensitive and painful. Procedural pain is the discomfort associated with medical or nursing care interventions. In burn patients, this type of pain is a major psychological burden and is often associated with a preemptive phase of severe anxiety and anticipatory distress "anticipatory pain" before the actual procedure or intervention actually occurs. In these cases, even common interventions, such as switching the side of patient recumbency, can induce excruciating breakthrough pain.

Aggressive analgesia must be provided at admission and maintained during the course of hospitalization, tapered to the patient's needs. In severe cases, preemptive analgesia should be provided before any even seemingly minor medical intervention to avoid and control procedural and breakthrough pain. Agents commonly used to treat burn pain include opioid analgesics, nonopioid analgesics, local anesthetics, and anxiolytics.[31]

Opioid analgesia represents the mainstay for burn pain. Constant rate infusions are effective at providing near-constant plasma levels of analgesics and maintaining control of background pain. Intermittent boluses are useful as a preemptive strategy or for control of sudden breakthrough pain.[32]

Nonopioid analgesics, such as dexmedetomidine and ketamine, provide effective analgesia and sedation, and are helpful for burn debridement and dressing changes. In resuscitated patients, dexmedetomidine provides effective sedation and analgesia for minor procedures and for control of breakthrough pain.[33,34] Ketamine as intermittent boluses (0.5-1 mg/kg) or a constant rate infusion (5–10 μg/kg/min) has a strong synergistic effect with opioid analgesics and its use in burn patients is particularly recommended for refractory and procedural pain.[35,36] Use of nonsteroidal antiinflammatory drugs is not recommended in the acute setting, because in the hemodynamically unstable patient there is a high risk of negative effects on renal blood flow autoregulation. They provide mild analgesia and are best suited as adjunctive option to treat burn pain once the patient has fully regained cardiovascular homeostasis.

Regional anesthesia and specifically nerve blockade has a strong synergic effect with systemic analgesia, allowing to reduce opioid use substantially. Regional anesthesia is particularly useful for burn pain relief involving the extremities and in human patients represents standard of care in this setting.[37] The most common nerve structures accessible for a nerve block include the brachial plexus, the sciatic nerve, and the femoral nerve. Ultrasound guidance is extremely helpful for accurate identification of the target nerve structure.[38]

Anxiety is known to exacerbate acute pain and the use of anxiolytic drugs in combination with analgesics is recommended in patients requiring multiple interventions and prolonged hospitalization. This practice is particularly useful for wound care owing to the anticipatory anxiety experienced before and during such procedures.[39] In the authors' experience, trazodone (3-5 mg/kg) administered by mouth twice daily seems to be a very suitable option for this purpose in injured dogs, with minimal to no negative cardiovascular effect.

Burn patients have metabolic, respiratory, cardiovascular, and thermoregulatory abnormalities that are associated with increased anesthetic risk. Severe burn injury also inconsistently alters the pharmacokinetic and pharmacodynamic response to many drugs with secondary abnormal responses to anesthetic agents and muscle relaxants. As an example, propofol clearance and volume of distribution are increased in burn patients and depolarizing muscle relaxant can be associated with the occurrence of life-threatening hyperkalemia.[40] Thus, intensive anesthetic monitoring and minimizing the duration of any anesthetic procedure in severe burn patients is highly recommended.

INTENSIVE CARE MANAGEMENT

After initial stabilization of the burn patient, maintenance of organ perfusion, respiratory monitoring and support, and pain control are ongoing priorities in intensive care, with the addition of control of burn-associated hypermetabolic syndrome, gastric ulcer prophylaxis, prevention of infection, and thromboprophylaxis. Nutritional support, effective pain management, and early burn wound management along with selected pharmacologic strategies are effective at blunting and modulating the severity of the hypermetabolic response to injury.[41]

Hypermetabolic Syndrome

Profound metabolic changes occur in patients suffering from severe burns. The hypermetabolic syndrome in burn patients is characterized by hyperdynamic circulatory, physiologic, and catabolic responses. A marked and sustained increase in the release of catecholamines, glucocorticoids, glucagon, and other hormones leads to an acute hypermetabolic state. Proinflammatory cytokines, neutrophil adherence complexes, reactive oxygen species, coagulation, and complement cascades have been implicated in regulating this response to burn injury.[42,43]

Two distinct and sequential phases of metabolic dysregulation are described. The ebb phase occurs within the first 48 hours of injury. This phase is characterized by decreased cardiac output and vasodilation, as well as impaired glucose tolerance and hyperglycemia. The flow phase follows and represents a rapid increase in metabolism over the first few days after injury. This phase is associated with hyperdynamic circulation with increased heart rate and cardiac output, and the development of insulin resistance.[42] The metabolic rate increases proportionally with burn size and patients with 20% TBSA burns commonly develop significant hypermetabolism.[44] This response can be sustained for up to 12 months after severe burn injuries and it is associated with significant changes in energy substrate metabolism. Both increased glucose and insulin fail to suppress hepatic glucose release, contributing to persistent hyperglycemia.[45] Catecholamines enhance hepatic glycogenolysis and impair glucose use by inducing peripheral insulin resistance via the downregulation of GLUT4 in skeletal muscle.[27]

Severe burn considerably reduces the ability of the body to use lipids as an energy source by suppression of beta-oxidation and skeletal muscle becomes the primary source of substrate for glucose production, which leads to marked decrease of lean body mass within days after burn injury.[46,47]

Nutritional Support

Nutritional support represents one of the most important interventions in the management of patients severe burn injury. The primary goal of nutritional support after severe burns is to meet the distinctive energy and nutritional demands of burn injury patients and mitigate the severity of hypermetabolism.[48]

In patients with a 20% TBSA burn, initiating nutritional support in the form of enteral feeding within 24 to 48 hours is suggested.[49] Enteral nutrition is the preferred form of support in burn patients because it maintains the integrity of the intestinal mucosa and relative immunity, decreases the occurrence of gastroparesis, and is crucial to meet the energy and nutrients requirements.[50]

A nasogastric feeding tube should be placed in patients with a severe burn injury soon after initial stabilization. Enteral feedings are initiated at a low rate and increased to an established goal rate over the next 12 to 24 hours. Placement of a nasogastric tube allows early delivery of enteral nutrition and monitoring of gastric residual volumes, provides gastric decompression if needed, and initiates gastric ulcer prophylaxis.[51]

Parenteral nutrition is currently contraindicated in burn patients because it is associated with increased mortality.[52] Thus, every effort should be made to optimize delivery enterally. In human burn patients, morbidity was shown to be significantly reduced in patients who received enteral nutrition compared with those who received parenteral nutrition. Those who received enteral nutrition had significantly higher serum albumin levels and fewer hypoglycemic events, electrolyte abnormalities, pulmonary and septic complications, and lower mortality.[53]

Considering the specific and constantly mutating metabolic alterations secondary to burn injury, the authors highly recommend consulting with a veterinary nutritionist for the formulation and ongoing modifications of an appropriate enteral diet in every severe burn patient.

Gastric Ulcer Prophylaxis

Burn shock often results in mesenteric vasoconstriction predisposing to gastric distension, mucosal ulceration (so-called Curling's ulcer), and functional ileus. Burn patients are at very high risk of gastric ulceration and it is indicated to initiate gastric ulcer prophylaxis soon after admission.[54] There is no definitive agreement on the ideal drug and dosing regimen to reduce gastric secretion in critically ill dogs and cats; often, the choice is based on the available data in healthy animals.

Chemoprophylaxis

Patients with severe burns are often immunocompromised on the basis of altered neutrophil chemotaxis, lymphocyte dysfunction, and imbalance in the production of proinflammatory cytokines. Nonsuperficial burns also destroy the physical barrier to bacterial colonization, which facilitates spread to the dermis and through the lymphatics.[55–58] Once bacterial invasion occurs, organisms can proliferate in necrotic tissue, and can spread the infection via hematogenous route. Therefore, prophylaxis against infection with topical antibiotics is given to all patients with nonsuperficial burns. Topical chemoprophylaxis is typically maintained until wound epithelialization is complete. Classically, silver sulfadiazine is used and bacitracin or triple antibiotic ointments (eg, polymyxin B, neomycin) are good alternative topical antibiotic in this setting. More details about antibiotic choices are provided elsewhere in this article.[59]

The use of prophylactic systemic antibiotics remains controversial. A recent review found no benefit for systemic antibiotic prophylaxis in reducing the incidence of burn wound infection and the occurrence of sepsis.[60] Systemic antimicrobial therapy is obviously indicated for any patients with ongoing burn wound infection or evidence of sepsis.

Thromboprophylaxis

Inflammation and coagulation are heavily interlinked with one another. Severe burns are associated to massive release of proinflammatory mediators with severe consequences on coagulation homeostasis. The greatest risk for thrombosis is for patients with burns greater than 20% TBSA.[61] In general, thromboprophylaxis in burn patients does not differ from that of other patients treated in an intensive care unit setting. In human burn patients, it is recommended to initiate thromboprophylaxis upon admission to the intensive care unit.[62] No consensus or definitive guidelines are available on the ideal choice, initiation, and duration of thromboprophylaxis in critical small animal patients. Monitoring of the patient's coagulation profile with repeated assessment of platelet count, clotting times, serum fibrinogen concentration, and thromboelastography allow to titrate thromboprophylactic interventions to the specific patient needs.

WOUND MANAGEMENT
Hydrotherapy and Cleaning of Wound

Immediate hydrotherapy may be beneficial in the burn patient because it may help to reduce the formation of zones of coagulation, reduce formation of edema, increase the speed of reepithelialization, and improve pain control. Cool (12°C [54°F]) water or saline-soaked gauze can be applied over 15 to 30 minutes.[63] It is important that cold water or ice not be used, because there is the potential for vasoconstriction, hypothermia, and exacerbation of injury. Monitoring the rectal temperature is recommended to ensure hydrotherapy does not result in hypothermia, especially in patients with TBSA burns greater than 15%—the goal is to cool the wound, but not the patient.[10] Warmed intravenous fluids, use of insulating blankets, and early dressing of damaged skin surface may be used to ensure adequate core temperature. The patient should not be immersed in a tub of water, because there is the potential for fecal fallout that could contaminate the delicate burn wound.[64] Irrigation may also be beneficial in removing debris embedded within the wound.[10] The addition of mineral oil to hydrotherapy may help with the removal of tar, if present.[63] Disinfectants could inhibit the healing process; thus, the use of saline or mild soap and water for cleaning of wounds is earning favor.[10]

Escharectomy

Eschars are stiff areas of dermis that form on the surface of partial thickness and full-thickness burn wounds. Definitive classification of the burn can be challenging until they are removed because they can obstruct visualization of the full depth of the injury. Eschars can cause pain, because the patient moving causes pulling of the rigid eschar on tender, damaged skin. Circumferential wounds with eschars can lead to impaired chest excursion or limb ischemia owing to constriction.[64,65] Escharotomy may be performed to improve distal circulation in circumferential extremity wounds.[63] There is an increased risk of infection with eschars, because they can create a protected environment for bacterial growth and impair dermal protective mechanisms.[66,67] Early removal of the eschar is recommended to prevent these complications, as well as allow application of medications directly to the wound, providing better drug penetration.

Topical Antibiotics

Topical antibiotics are recommended to reduce infection of the vulnerable, nonsuperficial burn wound (**Table 6**). Silver sulfadiazine is commonly used, providing broad-spectrum bactericidal effects, as well as effects on yeast and molds. Human studies have demonstrated the benefit of silver sulfadiazine on burn wounds and its limited systemic effects are appealing; however, it may delay separation of the eschar.[68] Medical grade honey is another broad-spectrum option with limited systemic effects, helping to promote better wound strength and granulation tissue formation with less wound contraction.[69] There are no data, however, showing the benefit of honey on burn wounds and local tissue sensitivity is possible. Broad-spectrum mafenide may be used before an escharectomy, because it has better eschar penetration, although it may be painful on application.[68] Bacitracin, polymyxin B, and neomycin may also be considered. After cleaning of wounds and application of antibiotics, a nonadherent mesh gauze or other wound dressing should be applied.

Table 6
Topical antibiotic options for burn wounds

Drug	Spectrum	Advantages	Disadvantages
Silver sulfadiazine	• Gram positive • Gram negative • Yeast, molds • MRSA • Molds • Yeast	• Study benefit • Slow and sustained release • Limited systemic effects • Eschar penetration	• Local hypersensitivity • May delay eschar separation • Argyria
Honey	• Gram positive • Gram negative • MRSA	• Decreased wound contracture and hypergranulation • Improved strength of wound • Improved rate of healing	• Local hypersensitivity
Mafenide acetate	• Gram positive • Gram negative • Limited MRSA effect	• Good penetration of eschar	• Local hypersensitivity • Painful when applied

Each has specific advantages and disadvantages that should be taken into consideration for the individual patient.
Abbreviation: MRSA, methicillin-resistant *Staphylococcus aureus.*

REFERENCES

1. Hettiaratchy S, Dziewulski P. ABC of burns: pathophysiology and types of burns. BMJ 2004;328:1427.
2. Ryan C, Schoenfeld D, Thorpe W, et al. Objective estimates of the probability of death from burn injuries. N Engl J Med 1998;338(6):362–6.
3. Bloemsma G, Dokter J, Boxma H, et al. Mortality and causes of death in a burn centre. Burns 2008;34:1103.
4. Mertens D, Jenkins M, Warden G. Outpatient burn management. Nurs Clin North Am 1997;32(2):343–64.
5. Baxter C. Management of burn wounds. Dermatol Clin 1993;11(4):709–14.
6. Wachtel T, Berry C, Wachtel E, et al. The inter-rater reliability of estimating the size of burns from various burn area chart drawings. Burns 2000;26(2):156–70.
7. Monafo W. Initial management of burns. N Engl J Med 1996;335(21):1581–6.
8. Orgill D. Excision and skin grafting of thermal burns. N Engl J Med 2009;360(9): 893–901.
9. Gomez M, Wong D, Stewart T, et al. The FLAMES score accurately predicts mortality risk in burn patients. J Trauma 2008;65:636–45.
10. Atiyeh B, Barret J, Dahai H, et al. International best practice guidelines: effective skin and wound management of non-complex burns. London, UK: Wounds International; 2014. p. 1–23.
11. Roberts G, Lloyd M, Parker M, et al. The Baux score is dead. Long live the Baux score: a 27-year retrospective cohort study of mortality at a regional burns service. J Trauma Acute Care Surg 2012;72(1):251–6.
12. Ipaktchi K, Arbabi S. Advances in burn critical care. Crit Care Med 2006;34:S239.
13. Cancio L. Airway management and smoke inhalation injury in the burn patient. Clin Plast Surg 2009;36:555.
14. Toon M, Maybauer M, Greenwood J, et al. Management of the acute smoke inhalation injury. Crit Care Resusc 2010;12:53.

15. Thompson J, Marrs T. Hydroxocobalamin in cyanide poisoning. Clin Toxicol 2012; 50(10):875–85.

16. Greenhalgh D. Steroids in the treatment of smoke inhalation injury. J Burn Care Res 2009;30(1):165–9.

17. Desai M, Mlcak R, Richardson J, et al. Reduction in mortality in pediatric patients with inhalation injury with aerosolized heparin/N-acetylcysteine therapy. J Burn Care Rehabil 1998;19:210.

18. Murakami K, McGuire R, Cox R, et al. Heparin nebulization attenuates acute lung injury in sepsis following smoke inhalation in sheep. Shock 2002;18:236.

19. Williams F, Herndon D, Suman O, et al. Changes in cardiac physiology after severe burn injury. J Burn Care Res 2011;32:269.

20. Chung K, Wolf S, Cancio L, et al. Resuscitation of severely burned military casualties: fluid begets more fluid. J Trauma 2009;67:231.

21. Klein M, Hayden D, Elson C, et al. The association between fluid administration and outcome following major burn: a multicenter study. Ann Surg 2007;245:622.

22. Blumetti J, Hunt J, Arnoldo B, et al. The Parkland formula under fire: is the criticism justified? J Burn Care Res 2008;29:180.

23. Theron A, Bodger O, Williams D. Comparison of three techniques using the Parkland formula to aid fluid resuscitation in adult burns. Emerg Med 2014;31:730.

24. Perel P, Roberts I. Colloids versus crystalloids for fluid resuscitation in critically ill patients. Cochrane Database Syst Rev 2012;(6):CD000567.

25. Bunn F, Roberts I, Tasker R, et al. Hypertonic versus near isotonic crystalloid for fluid resuscitation in critically ill patients. Cochrane Database Syst Rev 2004;(3):CD002045.

26. Wise R, Jacobs J, Pilate S, et al. Incidence and prognosis of intra-abdominal hypertension and abdominal compartment syndrome in severely burned patients: Pilot study and review of the literature. Anaesthesiol Intensive Ther 2016;48:95.

27. Dulhunty J, Boots R, Rudd M, et al. Increased fluid resuscitation can lead to adverse outcomes in major-burn injured patients, but low mortality is achievable. Burns 2008;34:1090.

28. Mustonen K, Vuola J. Acute renal failure in intensive care burn patients (ARF in burn patients). J Burn Care Res 2008;29:227.

29. Holm C, Tegeler J, Mayr M, et al. Effect of crystalloid resuscitation and inhalation injury on extravascular lung water: clinical implications. Chest 2002;121(6):1956.

30. Patterson D, Hofland H, Epsey K, et al. Pain management. Burns 2004;30:A10.

31. Abdi S, Zhou Y. Management of pain after burn injury. Curr Opin Anaesthesiol 2002;15(5):563–7.

32. Richardson P, Mustard L. The management of pain in the burns unit. Burns 2009; 35(7):921–36.

33. Lin H, Faraklas I, Sampson C, et al. Use of dexmedetomidine for sedation in critically ill mechanically ventilated pediatric burn patients. J Burn Care Res 2011; 32(1):98–103.

34. Walker J, Maccallum M, Fischer C, et al. Sedation using dexmedetomidine in pediatric burn patients. J Burn Care Res 2006;27(2):206–10.

35. McGuinness SK, Wasiak J, Cleland H, et al. A systematic review of ketamine as an analgesic agent in adult burn injuries. Pain Med 2011;12(10):1551–8.

36. Owens VF, Palmieri TL, Comroe CM, et al. Ketamine: a safe and effective agent for painful procedures in the pediatric burn patient. J Burn Care Res 2006; 27(2):211–6 [discussion: 217].

37. Cuignet O, Mbuyamba J, Pirson J. The long-term analgesic efficacy of a single-shot fascia iliac compartment block in burn patients undergoing skin-grafting procedures. J Burn Care Rehabil 2005;26(5):409–15.

38. Shteynberg A, Riina LH, Glickman LT, et al. Ultrasound guided lateral femoral cutaneous nerve (LFCN) block: safe and simple anesthesia for harvesting skin grafts. Burns 2013;39(1):146–9.

39. Vulink N, Figee M, Denys D. Review of atypical antipsychotics in anxiety. Eur Neuropsychopharmacol 2011;21(6):429–49.

40. Han T, Greenblatt D, Martyn J. Propofol clearance and volume of distribution are increased in patients with major burns. J Clin Pharmacol 2009;49(7):768–72.

41. Atiyeh B, Gunn S, Dibo S. Metabolic implications of severe burn injuries and their management: a systematic review of the literature. World J Surg 2008;32(8): 1857–69.

42. Grundy SM, Brewer HB, Cleeman JI, et al. Definition of metabolic syndrome: report of the National Heart, Lung, and Blood Institute/American Heart Association conference on scientific issues related to definition. Circulation 2004; 109(3):433–8.

43. Jeschke MG, Barrow RE, Herndon DN. Extended hypermetabolic response of the liver in severely burned pediatric patients. Arch Surg 2004;139(6):641–7.

44. Jeschke MG, Mlcak RP, Finnerty CC, et al. Burn size determines the inflammatory and hypermetabolic response. Crit Care 2007;11(4):R90.

45. Wolfe RR, Herndon DN, Jahoor F, et al. Effect of severe burn injury on substrate cycling by glucose and fatty acids. N Engl J Med 1987;317(7):403–8.

46. Hart DW, Wolf SE, Mlcak R, et al. Persistence of muscle catabolism after severe burn. Surgery 2000;128(2):312–9.

47. Cree MG, Aarsland A, Herndon DN, et al. Role of fat metabolism in burn trauma-induced skeletal muscle insulin resistance. Crit Care Med 2007;35(9 Suppl): S476–83.

48. Herndon DN, Tompkins RG. Support of the metabolic response to burn injury. Lancet 2004;363(9424):1895–902.

49. McClave SA, Martindale RG, Vanek VW, et al. Guidelines for the provision and assessment of nutrition support therapy in the adult critically ill patient: society of critical care medicine (SCCM) and American Society for Parenteral and Enteral Nutrition (A.S.P.E.N.). JPEN J Parenter Enteral Nutr 2009;33(3):277–316.

50. Prelack K, Dylewski M, Sheridan RL. Practical guidelines for nutritional management of burn injury and recovery. Burns 2007;33(1):14–24.

51. Mosier MJ, Pham TN, Klein MB, et al. Early enteral nutrition in burns: compliance with guidelines and associated outcomes in a multicenter study. J Burn Care Res 2011;32(1):104–9.

52. Herndon DN, Barrow RE, Stein M, et al. Increased mortality with intravenous supplemental feeding in severely burned patients. J Burn Care Rehabil 1989;10(4): 309–13.

53. Basaran O, Uysal S, Kesik E, et al. Comparison of frequency of complications in burn patients receiving enteral versus parenteral nutrition. Burns 2007;33S:S44.

54. Choi YH, Lee JH, Shin JJ, et al. A revised risk analysis of stress ulcers in burn patients receiving ulcer prophylaxis. Clin Exp Emerg Med 2015;2(4):250–5.

55. Stanojcic M, Chen P, Xiu F, et al. Impaired immune response in elderly burn patients: new insights into the immune-senescence phenotype. Ann Surg 2016; 264(1):195–202.

56. Bjerknes R, Vindenes H, Laerum OD. Altered neutrophil functions in patients with large burns. Blood Cells 1990;16(1):127–41 [discussion: 142–3].

57. Schwacha MG, Ayala A, Chaudry IH. Insights into the role of gammadelta T lymphocytes in the immunopathogenic response to thermal injury. J Leukoc Biol 2000;67(5):644–50.
58. Peter FW, Schuschke DA, Barker JH, et al. The effect of severe burn injury on proinflammatory cytokines and leukocyte behavior: its modulation with granulocyte colony-stimulating factor. Burns 1999;25(6):477–86.
59. Avni T, Levcovich A, Ad-El DD, et al. Prophylactic antibiotics for burns patients: systematic review and meta-analysis. BMJ 2010;340:c241.
60. Barajas-Nava L, Lopez-Alcalde J, Roque i Figuls M, et al. Antibiotic prophylaxis for preventing burn wound infection. Cochrane Database Syst Rev 2013;(6):CD008738.
61. Satahoo SS, Parikh PP, Naranjo D, et al. Are burn patients really at risk for thrombotic events? J Burn Care Res 2015;36(1):100–4.
62. Glas GJ, Levi M, Schultz MJ. Coagulopathy and its management in patients with severe burns. J Thromb Haemost 2016;14(5):865–74.
63. Rice P, Orgill D. Emergency care of moderate and severe thermal burns in adults. Alphen aan den Rijn, The Netherlands: Wolters Kluwer; 2016.
64. Latenser B. Critical care of the burn patient: the first 48 hours. Crit Care Med 2009;37(10):2819–26.
65. Sheridan R. Burns. In: Fink M, Abraham E, Vincent J, et al, editors. Textbook of critical care. 5th edition. Philadelphia: Elsevier Saunders; 2005. p. 2065–75.
66. Bishop J. Burn wound assessment and surgical management. Crit Care Nurs Clin North Am 2004;16(1):145–77.
67. Desanti L. Pathophysiology and current management of burn injury. Adv Skin Wound Care 2005;18(6):323–32.
68. Johnson R, Richard R. Partial-thickness burns: identification and management. Adv Skin Wound Care 2003;16(4):178–85.
69. Rozaini M, Zuki A, Noordin M, et al. The effect of different types of honey on tensile strength evaluation of burn wound tissue healing. J Appl Res Vet Med 2004; 2(4):290–6.

Management of Radiation Side Effects to the Skin

Tracy Gieger, DVM*, Michael Nolan, DVM, PhD

KEYWORDS

- Desquamation • Fibrosis • Cutaneous reaction • Radiation dermatitis • Erythema

KEY POINTS

- Radiation therapy (RT) is commonly used in the management of oncologic patients and owners must be counseled about potential side effects and their management before treatment.
- Acute radiation side effects to the skin occur during and immediately after a course of RT; are typically mild to moderate; and include epilation, erythema, dry and moist desquamation, and dermatitis.
- Late or chronic radiation side effects to the skin occur months to several years post-RT and include chronic dermatitis, leukotrichia, fibrosis, and ulceration.
- Careful radiation treatment planning and management of acute side effects are essential to prevent ongoing sequelae post-RT.
- There is no consensus regarding the best practice for management of acute radiation-induced dermatitis, and treatments may include oral or topical steroids, nonsteroidals, antibiotics, and barrier protectants.

INTRODUCTION

Radiation therapy (RT) is an essential component for management of many cancers and is becoming increasingly accessible to pet owners.[1] Veterinary health care professionals (including radiation and medical oncologists, veterinary technicians and radiation therapists, and dermatologists) must counsel owners about the potential side effects of RT, including the likelihood of occurrence and severity of the side effects, showing on the patient the sites where these effects are likely to be seen, and the anticipated management (and potential costs) of these effects. For most veterinary patients treated with RT, radiation side effects are mild and self-limiting; however, appropriate management of these side effects is essential to try to prevent chronic sequelae and the need for ongoing wound care.

Disclosure: The authors have nothing to disclose.
Department of Clinical Sciences, North Carolina State University, 1060 William Moore Drive, Raleigh, NC 27607, USA
* Corresponding author.
E-mail address: tlgieger@ncsu.edu

Vet Clin Small Anim 47 (2017) 1165–1180
http://dx.doi.org/10.1016/j.cvsm.2017.06.004
0195-5616/17/© 2017 Elsevier Inc. All rights reserved.

The skin is the dose-limiting organ for many sites in the body treated with RT and is the tissue most likely to experience side effects.[2] In most cases, external beam RT (EBRT) delivered with a linear accelerator is used to treat veterinary patients and is the cause of radiation-induced side effects; therefore, this article focuses on the definition of side effects resulting from EBRT and their management. The Veterinary Radiation Therapy Oncology Group published a document defining acute and late radiation-induced side effects of the skin and other organs (**Table 1**),[3] which is useful for documentation of side effects for clinical patients and to add objectivity to the study of side effects in prospective studies. Another study expanded this system to include the extent (focal vs generalized) of affected tissue.[4]

ACUTE RADIATION-INDUCED DERMATITIS

Acute radiation-induced dermatitis (ARID) develops in most patients receiving definitive-intent fractionated RT, and can cause pain, pruritus, and even treatment delays that could compromise the oncologic outcome.[4,5] Common manifestations of ARID include epilation, erythema, dry desquamation, and moist desquamation.[6] These effects are seen in the radiation field at sites of both entrance and exit dose. In dogs, generalized erythema (a blanchable pink hue) and epilation are commonly the first signs of ARID and are seldom associated with measurable discomfort. This effect is followed by dry desquamation, dyspigmentation (freckling and diffuse color changes), and scaling of the skin, which can be associated with pruritus. Moist desquamation with associated edema, erythema, and exudate follows as treatment progresses, and tends to be worse along scars if they are included in the radiation field. When acute changes do not resolve, they can result in consequential late effects (persistent, nonhealing acute radiation dermatitis). Various treatments, including pain management, are indicated to prevent self-trauma and to promote healing.

In dogs treated with commonly prescribed fractionated radiation protocols that consist of daily (Monday to Friday with breaks on weekends and holidays) treatments (called fractions) over a 15-day to 20-day regimen, these effects typically start about halfway through a radiation protocol and can worsen in the 1 to 2 weeks after the completion of treatment before they start to improve (**Fig. 1**).[4] Epidermal regeneration occurs in the 3 to 5 weeks after RT with complete healing within 1 to 3 months.[2,6] For treatment regimens consisting of once-weekly or twice-weekly treatments or a low total number of treatments, ARID may be minimal or not clinically observable. In contrast, patients receiving hyperfractionated radiation protocols (>1 radiation treatment per day) are likely to have more severe ARID. Anecdotally, cat skin is more

Table 1			
Veterinary Radiation Therapy Oncology Group morbidity scoring scheme for skin/hair			
Grade 0	Grade 1	Grade 2	Grade 3
Acute Effects			
No change over baseline	Erythema, dry desquamation, alopecia/epilation	Patchy moist desquamation without edema	Confluent moist desquamation
Late Effects			
None	Alopecia, hyperpigmentation, leukotrichia	Asymptomatic induration (fibrosis)	Severe induration causing physical impairment, necrosis

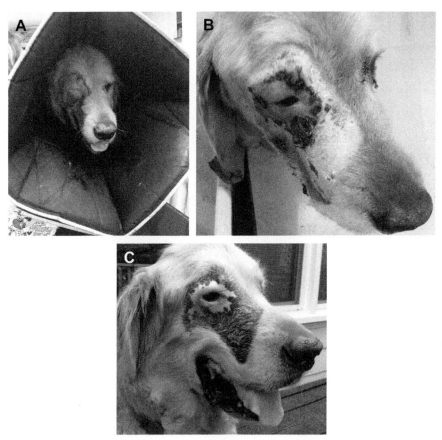

Fig. 1. Severe periocular ARID at the end of (*A*) 1 month, (*B*) 2 months, and (*C*) 4 months after treatment of an incompletely excised maxillary sarcoma. An intensity-modulated radiation therapy (IMRT) plan was used, which allowed the globe of the right eye to be spared more than the skin.

resistant to radiation-induced side effects, and acute effects are typically limited to epilation, erythema, and dry desquamation (**Fig. 2**).

Modern veterinary radiation oncology also includes the use of stereotactic RT (SRT), in which treatments consist of 1 to 5 daily treatments given during a single week, with large doses of radiation given per treatment.[7–9] Unlike conventional fractionated radiation treatment fields, which consist of a scar plus a margin of surrounding tissue to account for microscopic disease and patient interfraction and intrafraction motion, SRT involves the treatment of a well-defined, bulky tumor target with minimal (scatter) dose to surrounding (normal) tissues. The use of SRT has changed the skin toxicity profile in veterinary patients considerably. Acute toxicities are typically minimal because of low doses of radiation to normal tissues surrounding the tumor, and may consist of epilation or erythema that is seen in the 1 to 2 weeks after SRT is completed. Late or chronic side effects to the skin/mucosa, such as nasocutaneous (**Fig. 3**) or oronasal fistulas (following treatment of an intranasal or oral tumor) or full-thickness ulcerations over a treated bone (for primary appendicular bone tumors; **Fig. 4**) anecdotally occur earlier posttreatment than with traditional

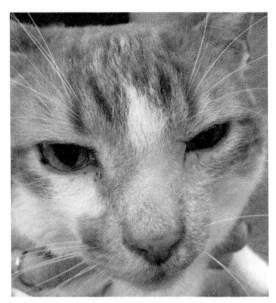

Fig. 2. Mild ARID seen in a cat at the end of fractionated RT for a nasal tumor.

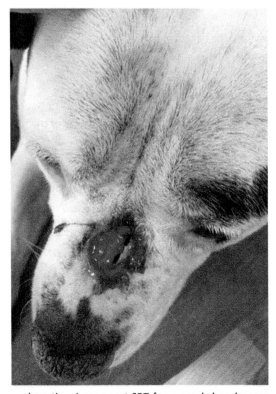

Fig. 3. Full-thickness ulceration 1 year post-SRT for a nasal chondrosarcoma.

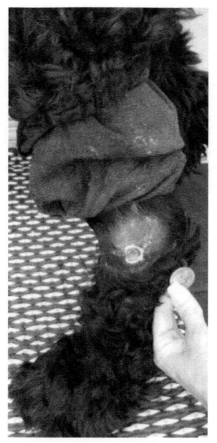

Fig. 4. Nonhealing full-thickness skin ulcer on the hock of a dog post-SRT for an osteosarcoma. (*Courtesy of* Dr Susan LaRue, Colorado State University, Fort Collins, CO.)

fractionated RT, which consists of lower daily doses of radiation delivered over a period of weeks.

Intensity-modulated RT (IMRT) planning techniques can be used to decrease the dose of radiation to the skin in some cases.[7] SRT treatments are frequently planned using IMRT, which is a computer-based treatment plan created with specialized software that allows the dose to be modulated across a treatment field (sometimes referred to as dose painting). Various technologies can be used to plan and deliver IMRT. With this type of RT planning, the skin is contoured as a separate organ (typically defined as 2-mm thickness inside of the body contour) and dose constraints can be made against the skin. For example, at our institution, the planning goal for the skin dose for a nasal tumor being treated with SRT in 3 daily 10-Gy fractions (total radiation dose to the tumor, 30 Gy) is less than 1 cm^3 of the total volume of skin greater than or equal to 24 Gy and to have no full thickness of skin at that dose (**Fig. 5**). The rapid dose falloff between the tumor and skin allows high-dose treatment of the tumor with skin sparing. In cases in which scars on the skin and adjacent subcutaneous tissues are being treated with full-course fractionated RT, IMRT planning can also be used to spare the

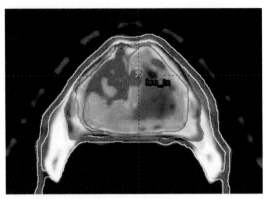

Fig. 5. Cross-sectional image from an IMRT plan from a dog being treated with SRT for a nasal tumor. The dose in color wash shows all structures receiving greater than or equal to 24 Gy. The skin (*yellow contour*) receives less than 24 Gy (dose to the tumor is ≥30 Gy).

skin to some degree, such as using modulation to reduce so-called hot spots in the skin.

Risk Factors for Development of Acute Radiation-induced Dermatitis

Reported risk factors for increasing incidence and severity of ARID in humans include larger radiation fields (larger exposed surface area), preexisting skin disease, smoking, concurrent connective tissue diseases such as systemic lupus, concurrent infectious diseases such as human immunodeficiency virus, and genetic factors.[6] Persons with ataxia telangiectasia, a rare autosomal recessive disorder resulting from mutations in both copies of the *ATM* gene, are predisposed to develop severe cutaneous complications after RT. Other syndromes, such as Gorlin syndrome (development of multiple basal cell carcinomas and increased radiosensitivity), chromosomal breakage syndromes, and disorders characterized by defects in DNA repair such as xeroderma pigmentosum, may also increase the risk of severe acute and late radiation side effects in people and are poorly characterized in veterinary patients.

In the single prospective veterinary study describing ARID and its treatment,[4] factors such as coat color, breed of dog, size of the radiation field, proportion of the radiation field with pigmented skin, and tumor location were not prognostic for the incidence or severity of ARID; however, this study represented only 22 dogs with heterogeneous skin and hair coat characteristics and tumor sites. Anecdotally, ARID is typically more severe when radiation fields include skin folds, nails and footpads, and inguinal and perianal skin (**Fig. 6**). Facial skin-fold dermatitis during and after RT is common in breeds such as English bulldogs and pugs, especially when they have preexisting skin disease before RT. The footpads may slough off when included in a radiation field, leaving behind a smooth, shiny pad that must be protected while it is healing (**Fig. 7**). Nails may also slough during or after RT, and the nails that regrow are often brittle; owners should be counseled that the affected nails should be kept trimmed, and a sanding tool may be the most effective way to keep the nails short. In patients with preexisting sun damage (eg, sunbathing dogs with ventral abdominal skin changes such as actinic keratosis), ARID may increase in severity compared with nonaffected dogs. Alopecia tends to have a faster onset and may be more likely to be permanent in dogs such as poodles with anagen-phase hair follicles. In many dogs with white or pink skin, the severity of ARID is worse than in dogs with pigmented skin.

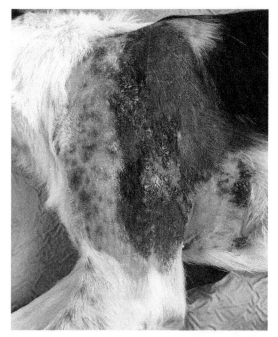

Fig. 6. Grade 3 ARID of the axillary region at the completion of a fractionated RT protocol (54 Gy in 18 daily fractions).

Pathophysiology of Acute Radiation-induced Dermatitis

ARID is a complex process resulting from impairment of functional stem cells, endothelial cell changes, inflammation, and epidermal cell apoptosis and necrosis.[2,5] The skin functional unit (SFU) consists of a microvessel with associated epidermis and dermis. During RT, the dose response of the SFU defines the dose response of the skin.[2] In a clinical model of swine skin in which a total radiation dose of 60 Gy was administered in 30 daily fractions over a 40-day period (Monday to Friday with weekends off), no histologic change was detected until doses of 20 to 25 Gy were delivered, when a loss of basal cell density occurred with a nadir around day 50 before rebounding. The surviving basal cells can provide sustained activity and provide epithelial regeneration of large areas of skin, with a typical turnover time of about 30 days from basal cell loss to replacement (paralleling the clinical healing time of ARID).[2,5] The effects to the microvasculature during this period are not well characterized. Endothelial cell proliferation has not been observed, so it is thought that blood vessels are lost without replacement. Remaining blood vessels may shorten and become dilated over a period of months to years (telangiectasia).[2,5,6]

Effects of Fractionation Modifications on Acute Radiation-induced Dermatitis

Uncommonly in veterinary patients, gaps of a few days or more during fractionated RT can occur related to patient or client factors. Such prolongation of the RT protocol can result in a phenomenon of accelerated repopulation, in which basal cell repopulation is accelerated after a lag period,[2] resulting in an increase in the radiosensitivity of the surviving stem cells and a decrease in the time required for cells to repair sublethal radiation-induced DNA damage.

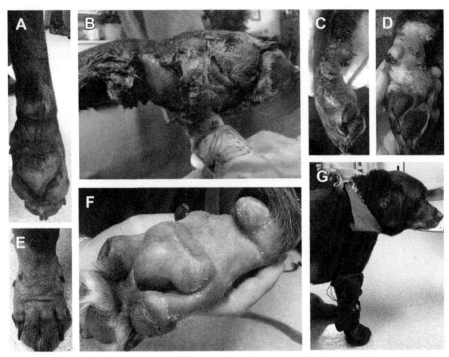

Fig. 7. Acute radiation dermatitis of the paw in a dog treated with a total dose of 54 Gy in 18 daily fractions. Progression from day 15 of RT (*A*), last day of RT (*B*), 4 days after completion (*C*) (note foot pad loss), 1 week after treatment (*D*), and 2 weeks after treatment with protective footwear shown (*E–G*).

MANAGEMENT OF ACUTE RADIATION-INDUCED DERMATITIS: OVERVIEW AND GOALS

In physician-based medicine, multiple clinical trials have been published on prevention and treatment of ARID. In one meta-analysis of 20 clinical trials involving more than 3000 patients assessing the use of topical agent therapy for either the prevention or treatment of ARID,[10] the conclusion was that no topical agent was superior in the prevention or treatment of ARID. In a publication of systematic reviews of all types of therapy for ARID,[11] conclusions were as follows: gentle skin and hair cleansing should not be restricted; topical steroids may improve dermatitis but are not recommended because they can cause skin thinning and increase bacterial infections; there were too few studies evaluating oral medications such as the radioprotectant amifostine, pentoxifylline (PTX), zinc supplements, and oral enzyme therapy to be conclusive about their efficacy; the use of moisture-vapor–permeable dressings may improve healing; and the use of modern radiotherapy techniques such as IMRT resulted in less severe ARID.

In contrast with the plethora of published information regarding management of ARID in people, only a single publication regarding the management of ARID exists in veterinary medicine.[12] A survey of 54 veterinary hospitals providing RT was conducted, and participants were asked to list all topical and systemic medications prescribed, whether every patient received the same treatment regimen or therapy was tailored to the individual, and when during the course of RT the medications were initiated. Treatments were considered prophylactic if initiated before the onset of moist desquamation and/or within the first 7 days of radiation treatment. There was wide variation in treatment recommendations, with only 7.5% of facilities using the same protocol. Two-thirds of facilities routinely used topical therapies, with aloe vera, 1% silver sulfadiazine cream, and chlorhexidine solution being the most commonly used. Topical steroids were used by 15% of practices, and compounds containing both steroids and antimicrobials were most commonly used. Some practices (28%) used products designed to restore the skin's barrier function, including gels and adhesive transparent films. Few (6%) practitioners used hydrotherapy to routinely rinse or soak the radiation site. Oral antibiotics and steroids were routinely prescribed in 78% and 57% of practices, respectively. Few practices routinely used nonsteroidal antiinflammatory drugs for control of ARID. Pain medication included tramadol (76%), gabapentin, fentanyl patches, and codeine plus acetaminophen in addition to oral steroids and/or nonsteroidals. About half of facilities used medications prophylactically, with the other group prescribing treatments after the onset of moist desquamation.

To more objectively assess the management of ARID, the same researchers who published the survey discussed earlier performed a prospective, randomized, double-blind, placebo-controlled study to compare prednisone versus placebo (sugar pill) on the clinical and histopathologic aspects of ARID.[4] Dogs with spontaneously arising tumors were treated postoperatively (in a microscopic disease setting) with a total dose of 48 Gy in daily 3-Gy fractions. A source-to-surface distance calculation method was used so that the maximum radiation dose was at the skin surface. The scar was treated with a 3-cm surrounding margin of normal tissue in all directions (deep and lateral) to account for microscopic disease extension. Dogs were treated with prednisone (0.5 mg/kg by mouth every 24 hours) or placebo starting on the first day of RT and continuing throughout the protocol, and weekly skin biopsies and cutaneous toxicity scoring were performed. A final examination and biopsy were performed 2 weeks after completion of RT. A published side effect scoring system[3] was expanded to include the extent of the reaction (focal vs generalized). Histopathology was performed to examine the skin for evidence of hyperkeratosis, follicular atrophy, hydropic degeneration, ulceration, and necrosis. In addition, skin cytology was performed to examine for evidence of bacterial and fungal skin infections. Eleven dogs were in each group and all completed therapy; tramadol was used in dogs that developed moist desquamation or discomfort associated with the area. Prednisone administration did not significantly decrease ARID severity, clinically or histopathologically, nor did it delay the onset of moist desquamation compared with placebo. Bacterial skin infections were diagnosed in 94% of the patients in this study (all treated with oral antibiotics) and *Malassezia* sp yeast infections were diagnosed in 46% (treated with oral ketoconazole or fluconazole), and the incidence did not vary between the groups (in humans, use of steroids in the management of ARID is implicated in predisposition to skin infections[6]). All infections resolved by the end of the study period. The results of this study did not support routine use of prednisone for prevention of ARID. It was acknowledged that future studies involving the use of prophylactic antibiotic therapy and/or monitoring for skin infections during therapy may also play a role in the management of ARID.

Pharmacologic Strategies in the Management of Acute Radiation-induced Dermatitis

Systemic medications

Oral pain medications are frequently indicated in veterinary patients receiving RT. There is some controversy about when to begin them; some radiation oncologists systematically begin pain medications at the start of, or halfway through, an RT regimen with a goal of prophylaxis of acute effects, whereas others wait until the onset of clinical signs of varying degrees.[4] Pain medications may include nonsteroidal antiinflammatory drugs, opioids, gabapentin, and N-methyl-D-aspartate inhibitors (amantadine). Oral steroids may be used to attempt to alleviate inflammation and itch in some cases. Transdermal fentanyl patches may also be useful in some patients, but only last for 3 to 4 days and can be costly. Antibiotics are used in patients with exudative wounds that appear to be infected; skin cytology may be useful in selection of antibiotics and can also be used to assess for secondary skin fungal infections.[12] Broad-spectrum antibiotics such as amoxicillin-clavulanate or cephalexin are commonly used until healing is complete; ongoing or resistant wound infections are uncommon.

Topical therapy
In humans, numerous topical therapies, including steroids, aloe vera, sucralfate, gentian violet, Biafine, Lipiderm cream, calendula ointment, and hyaluronic acid, have been used in the management of ARID,[10,11] although no consensus has been reached regarding superiority of any specific medication. In veterinary patients, the use of topical medications for the management of ARID is controversial and no single treatment has definitively been shown to improve symptoms.[12] Many veterinary radiation oncologists do not advocate the use of topical medications at all, whereas others routinely prescribe it for pets during and after completion of RT. Instructing pet owners to apply topical creams to an irradiated area that is uncomfortable for the pet can result in poor compliance and behavior changes in the pet, such as hiding or aggression when application of topical medications is attempted. Treatments such as antibacterial 1% silver sulfadiazine (generic) and emollient zinc oxide/calamine/menthol/lanolin (Calmoseptine cream, Calmo Manufacturing, Inc, Huntington Beach, CA) may be helpful in some settings; for example, if the perineum is being irradiated and the pet develops colitis and diarrhea, gentle daily cleaning of the area under anesthesia with water and chlorhexidine-soaked cotton sponges followed by topical application of an emollient lotion may help to keep the surrounding skin cleaner and moist. Because topical medications can act as a bolus material to the irradiated area (resulting in an increased skin dose), these therapies should only be applied after that day's treatment is complete, ideally while the pet is still under general anesthesia.

Nonpharmacologic Management Strategies for Acute Radiation-induced Dermatitis

Physical protection
The use of an e-collar is indicated for most dogs undergoing RT to prevent the patient from licking/biting the wound, which can delay healing and result in progression of ARID to consequential late effects. Counseling the owner before the initiation of RT about the eventual need for an e-collar is important. For many patients and pet owners, hard plastic see-through–type e-collars are intolerable because many dogs get caught in doorways and run into the owners with them. For these patients, use of more flexible (but still semirigid) cloth-type or inflatable-doughnut–type collars can be helpful (see **Fig. 1**A). In cats, routine use of e-collars is not recommended, and soft-sided e-collars suffice in most cats that begin to excessively groom their radiation sites. In areas of high friction, such as the axilla (see **Fig. 6**), ARID is likely to be more severe and may take longer to heal. In some cases, a loose-fitting T-shirt secured at the waist may provide protection, especially because some dogs scratch affected skin along the body wall or head/neck with their hind limbs and/or rub affected areas on the ground or on furniture.

During and after RT, irradiated skin should have minimal exposure to ultraviolet light, which can upregulate cytokine production and can serve as a cocarcinogen.[6]

For pets, avoiding sun exposure may necessitate lifelong use of sunscreen to the irradiated site (only applied to skin that is completely healed) or physical barriers such as hats or clothing designed for dogs (see **Fig. 7**).

Wound care

The use of wound dressings and bandages covering the irradiated area is not generally recommended because they may cause further adhesion of exudates onto the wound and also need to be changed regularly, which can be associated with discomfort because fibrinous exudates can become attached to adhesive dressings. When the foot or nails are included in the RT field, the use of a loose-fitting sock (held up with Velcro so that it can be easily removed) or a MediPaw boot (medivetproducts.com) may be the most useful means to protect the foot.

MANAGEMENT OF CHRONIC RADIATION DERMATITIS: OVERVIEW AND GOALS

Chronic or late radiation side effects can be seen several months to years after completion of RT. Permanent changes to the skin are common in veterinary patients after receiving RT but are typically mild and do not require treatment (**Fig. 8**). Alopecia, postinflammatory hypopigmentation and hyperpigmentation (dyspigmentation) of the skin, and leukotrichia are commonly seen, and typically persist (**Fig. 9**). Textural changes such as xerosis, scale, and hyperkeratosis are common,[6,13] and hair follicles and sebaceous glands may appear to be absent in the field. In dogs treated with RT in which the field includes the nasal planum, there is often development of diffuse, persistent hyperkeratosis of the nasal planum (**Fig. 10**). In dogs in which the entire circumference of the limb or tail is included in the radiation field, lymphedema may occur around and distal to the site. Fibrosis is characterized by progressive induration, edema formation, and thickening of the dermis and subcutaneous tissues[2] and can lead to breakdown of the skin with resultant ulcerations and infection that must be managed by a team consisting of radiation oncologists, soft tissue surgeons, and sometimes dermatologists.

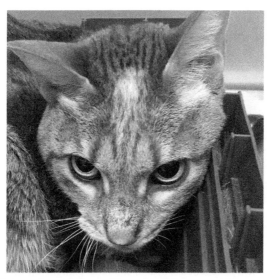

Fig. 8. Hair coat changes in a cat 6 months post-SRT for a nasal tumor.

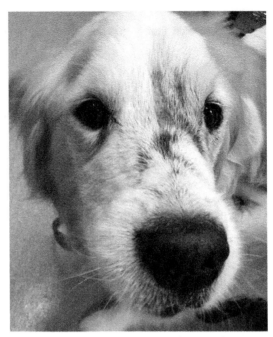

Fig. 9. Grade 1 late effects 1 year after completion of fractionated radiation therapy for a nasal tumor.

Chronic radiation dermatitis is poorly characterized in the veterinary literature. In a retrospective study of 51 dogs receiving greater than or equal to 48-Gy pelvic canal irradiation in fraction sizes ranging from 2.25 to 4 Gy for various tumors in the region, 7 dogs developed chronic skin ulcerations or draining tracts.[14] Dogs with perineal tumors (vs other pelvic canal locations) and those with larger radiation fields were at

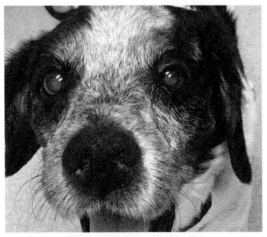

Fig. 10. Changes to the hair coat (leukotrichia) and nasal planum (diffuse dry crusting of the nasal planum) remain stable for more than 2 years post-SRT for a nasal tumor.

higher risk for developing these complications. The management of these wounds was not described, and no patient was reported to have been euthanized as a direct result of them.

Radiation protocols should be designed with the goal of minimizing the chances of late side effects because these conditions affect the patient's quality of life, add to the costs of treatment, and are difficult to manage clinically. Considerations by the radiation oncologist should include minimizing the dose/fraction, keeping the inter-fraction interval greater than or equal to 6 hours to allow for maximum sublethal DNA damage repair, avoidance of bolus to the skin (when possible), and making sure that field sizes are not larger than the intended target area to minimize normal tissue irradiation.[13,14] Sparing a strip of skin on the edge of the radiation field to avoid irradiating the entire circumference of a limb or tail may prevent lymphedema as a late effect.

Radiation-induced malignancies have been reported as a rare late effect in veterinary patients and can be seen in the skin or other tissues (bones) several months to years after RT.[14,15] In humans, irradiated skin has increased risks of developing basal cell carcinoma and other nonmelanoma skin cancers, which increases in white people and with radiation treatment at an earlier age.[6]

Pathophysiology of Chronic Radiation Dermatitis

Transforming growth factor beta (TGF-β) is considered the primary cytokine associated with the development of chronic radiation dermatitis, inducing tissue fibrosis via stimulating fibroblasts to secrete extracellular matrix proteins.[2,6,13,16] TGF-β is present in irradiated tissues in higher levels than in nonirradiated controls, and is considered part of the general response of cells to ionizing radiation. Radiation-induced endothelial cell damage activates components of the coagulation system, which in turn promote inflammation and cytokine overproduction. Thrombin may also modulate the synthesis of TGF-β and induce vascular endothelial permeability, inflammation, and tissue remodeling. Subsequent extracellular matrix accumulation, fibrosis, endothelial cell dysfunction, and increase in cytokine levels may further delay reepithelialization and cause vascular sclerosis. Fibroblasts may be permanently altered, causing dermal and subcutaneous atrophy (loss of fibrocytes and collagen reabsorption), contraction, and fibrosis. This long-lasting impairment can result in prolonged loss of integrity/wound strength in irradiated tissues.

Pharmacologic Strategies in the Management of Chronic Radiation Dermatitis

As is the case with ARID, there is no gold standard in the management of chronic radiation dermatitis in human or veterinary medicine, and treatments are largely symptomatic.[13]

PTX is a methylxanthine derivative that inhibits platelet aggregation, increases phagocytic activity of polymorphonuclear leukocytes and monocytes, and may antagonize the effects of TGF-β.[6,13,16] In a pig model, PTX had a significant antifibrotic effect and reversed radiation-induced fibrosis.[16] The combination of PTX and vitamin E (alpha-tocopherol acetate) may further downregulate TGF-β expression by myofibroblasts and may reverse the abnormal fibroblast phenotype that perpetuates fibrosis. The prophylactic use of PTX does not modify ARID or prevent lymphedema, but, for late effects, has been shown to decrease the incidence and severity of fibrosis and soft tissue necrosis. It also accelerated healing of soft tissue necrosis and reversed some late radiation injuries, including fibrosis. Other modalities that have been used in humans to treat chronic radiation-induced fibrosis include injectable liposomal superoxide dismutase and low-dose interferon gamma.[6]

Nonpharmacologic Strategies in the Management of Chronic Radiation Dermatitis

Hyperbaric oxygen therapy (HBOT) can induce neovascularization in irradiated tissue and reepithelialization of small areas of skin, as well as reducing pain, edema, erythema, and lymphedema, although it has not been shown to decrease radiation-induced fibrosis or telangiectasia.[6,17] Mechanisms of action in radiation-induced syndromes include modulation of platelet-derived growth factor beta receptors, increased resistance to infection via improved neutrophil function, and bacteriostatic effects. Although HBOT is not widely available to veterinary patients, its use should be considered in the management of chronic radiation-induced ulcers or fistulas.

SURGICAL CONSIDERATIONS ASSOCIATED WITH RADIOTHERAPY
Preoperative Versus Postoperative Radiation Therapy

Although postoperative RT is most commonly used in veterinary patients (treating a scar with a margin of surrounding tissue [typically 3–5 cm surrounding the scar and surgical site] to account for microscopic disease, intrafraction motion, and interfraction motion of the patient), preoperative RT may be elected in some cases. Preoperative RT is most commonly considered in cats with injection site sarcomas,[18] with the goal of treating the gross tumor and a margin of surrounding normal tissue to "sterilize" microscopic tumor extensions. Possible benefits of preoperative RT include a reduction in volume of normal tissue irradiated, improved oxygenation (vs a relatively hypoxic surgical bed), and lower RT dose. The lower total RT dose is acceptable because the relative biological effectiveness of RT improves in the absence of surgery-induced hypoxia, and without the increased tumor doubling time that occurs in tumor cells left behind after surgery. There have not been veterinary studies to date to determine the best regimen for preoperative RT.

Use of Cutaneous or Mucosal Flaps in Irradiated Tissues

In many tumor-bearing patients, use of both surgery and RT is indicated to try to attain the best outcome. In some cases, tumors are too large to be surgically removed and the associated wound closed, and cutaneous or mucosal flaps may assist with closure.[19] In pets treated with preoperative RT, there is concern that irradiated skin may not heal and flaps used to close the wound would not be effective. In a single published study of dogs treated with surgery involving a mucosal or cutaneous flap, groups of dogs included (1) dogs that had planned preoperative RT (N = 8), (2) dogs that had planned postoperative RT (N = 9), and (3) dogs in which flaps were used to manage either RT-associated complications or tumor recurrence after RT (N = 9). Most dogs (77%) had a complication of the flap, and 54% had 2 or more complications. Six dogs required another flap and 4 had unresolved complications. Flap complications were defined as necrosis, infection, dehiscence, and ulceration. Flaps that were used to manage a complication had a greater than 19 times higher risk of complication than planned flaps. There was no difference in complications between dogs with planned preoperative versus postoperative RT. Radiation protocols using 3 Gy/d 5 days a week had a lower risk of complications than those using 4 Gy on alternate days. Overall, in 85% of the dogs of the study, flaps were successful despite associated complications. (For additional insight regarding cutaneous flaps, see Laura C. Cuddy's article, "Wound Closure, Tension-Relieving Techniques, and Local Flaps," in this issue.)

ASSOCIATED SYNDROMES: RADIATION RECALL AND RADIATION SENSITIZATION
Radiation Sensitization

Radiation sensitizers are drugs given during or within 7 days before or after radiation, causing increased cellular damage and impaired repair.[6] Most commonly, these are chemotherapy drugs, but other medications such as antibiotics can also have radiosensitizing effects. In humans, methotrexate, taxanes, platinum drugs, and 5-fluorouracil have commonly been implicated as radiosensitizers.[2,6,13] In veterinary medicine, concurrent chemoradiation is not widely used and few publications describing it exist.[14,20] In one report, increased acute radiation toxicity (oral mucositis and hematologic toxicity) was seen in dogs and cats treated with gemcitabine in conjunction with RT for head and neck carcinomas.[20] Molecularly targeted therapies have been used as radiosensitizers in human head and neck cancers and may result in increased efficacy of radiotherapy protocols without increased normal tissue toxicity.[21]

Radiation Recall

Radiation recall is a phenomenon that can be seen at any time (days to years) after completion of RT and results from administration of a pharmacologic agent (typically a chemotherapy drug), and it creates an apparent recurrence of acute RT side effects that are sharply demarcated by the radiation field.[22] Note that not all patients that experience radiation recall had any type of ARID during therapy. Although the skin has been the primary site for radiation recall toxicity, instances in other organs have been reported as well. Severity can range from erythema to necrosis, ulceration, and hemorrhage, and histopathology consists of a nonspecific inflammatory infiltrate. The pathophysiology of this phenomenon is not well known but can include impaired cellular repair, gene mutation, epidermal skin cell inadequacy and depletion, drug hypersensitivity, cumulative direct DNA damage and oxidative stress, upregulation of cytokines, and vascular damage. In humans, use of doxorubicin, taxanes, actinomycin, gemcitabine, vinblastine, bleomycin, and others (including nonpharmacologic agents, such as sunlight) have been implicated in the occurrence of this rare syndrome.[2,22] Although there are no published instances of radiation recall in veterinary medicine, it has been seen by the authors. Treatment involves supportive care and withdrawal of the offending agent when possible.

FUTURE DIRECTIONS

Limitations in studying acute and late radiation side effects in veterinary medicine include lack of consistent long-term follow-up for treated patients and lack of an in-depth comprehensive toxicity scoring system that is used prospectively. At our institution, a prospective study is ongoing to establish a pain and behavior scoring system to attempt to establish a comprehensive, subjective, and objective evaluation of ARID-associated pain in patients receiving RT. Establishing evidence-based protocols for management of radiation-associated pain and acute and late toxicity will significantly affect veterinary patients undergoing RT.

REFERENCES

1. Farrelly J, McEntee MC. A survey of veterinary radiation facilities in 2010. Vet Radiol Ultrasound 2014;55(6):638–43.
2. Archambeau JO, Penzer R, Wasserman T. Pathophysiology of irradiated skin and breast. Int J Radiat Oncol Biol Phys 1995;31(5):1171–85.

3. Ladue T, Klein MK. Toxicity criteria of the Veterinary Radiation Therapy Oncology Group. Vet Radiol Ultrasound 2001;42:475–6.

4. Flynn AK, Lurie DM, Ward J, et al. The clinical and histopathological effects of prednisone on acute radiation-induced dermatitis in dogs: a placebo-controlled, randomized, double-blind, prospective clinical trial. Vet Dermatol 2007;18(4):217–26.

5. Parker RG, Juillard GJ. Skin: the basic model for relating dose, time, and fractionation. Front Radiat Ther Oncol 1988;22:53–61.

6. Hymes SR, Strom EA, Fife C. Radiation dermatitis: clinical presentation, pathophysiology, and treatment 2006. J Am Acad Dermatol 2006;54:28–46.

7. LaRue SM, Custis JT. Advances in veterinary radiation therapy. Vet Clin Small Anim 2014;44:909–23.

8. Glasser SA, Charney S, Dervisis N, et al. Use of an image-guided robotic radiosurgery system for the treatment of canine nonlymphomatous nasal tumors. J Am Anim Hosp Assoc 2016;50(2):96–104.

9. Farese JP, Milner R, Thompson MS, et al. Stereotactic radiosurgery for treatment of osteosarcoma involving the distal portions of the limbs in dogs. J Am Vet Med Assoc 2004;225(10):1567–72.

10. Zhang Y, Zhang S, Shao X. Topical agent therapy for prevention and treatment of radiodermatitis: a meta-analysis. Support Care Cancer 2013;21:1025–31.

11. Chan RJ, Larsen E, Chan P. Re-examining the evidence in radiation dermatitis management literature: an overview and critical appraisal of systematic reviews. Int J Radiat Oncol Biol Phys 2012;84(3):e357–62.

12. Flynn AK, Lurie DM. Canine acute radiation dermatitis, a survey of current management practices in North America. Vet Comp Oncol 2007;5(4):197–207.

13. Cooper JS, Fu K, Marks J, et al. Late effects of radiation therapy in the head and neck region. Int J Radiat Oncol Biol Phys 1995;31(5):1141–64.

14. Arthur JJ, Kleiter MM, Thrall DE, et al. Characterization of normal tissue complications in 51 dogs undergoing definitive pelvic region irradiation. Vet Radiol Ultrasound 2008;49(1):85–9.

15. Gillette SM, Gillette EL, Powers BE, et al. Radiation-induced osteosarcoma in dogs after external beam or intraoperative radiation therapy. Cancer Res 1990; 50:54–7.

16. Lefaix JL, Delanian S, Vozenin MC, et al. Striking regression of subcutaneous fibrosis induced by high doses of gamma rays using a combination of pentoxifylline and alpha-tocopherol: an experimental study. Int J Radiat Oncol Biol Phys 1999;43:839–47.

17. Kulikovsky M, Gil T, Messantes I, et al. Hyperbaric oxygen therapy for non-healing wounds. Isr Med Assoc J 2009;11:480–5.

18. Kobayashi T, Hauck ML, Dodge R, et al. Preoperative radiotherapy for vaccine-associated fibrosarcomas in 92 cats. Vet Radiol Ultrasound 2002;43(5):473–9.

19. Seguin B, McDonald DE, Kent MS, et al. Tolerance of mucosal flaps placed into a radiation therapy field in dogs. Vet Surg 2005;34:214–22.

20. LeBlanc AK, LaDue TA, Turrel JM, et al. Unexpected toxicity following use of gemcitabine as a radiosensitizer in head and neck carcinomas. Vet Radiol Ultrasound 2004;45(5):466–70.

21. Yamamoto VN, Thylur DS, Bauschard M, et al. Overcoming radioresistance in head and neck squamous cell carcinoma. Oral Oncol 2016;63:44–5.

22. Azria D, Magne N, Zouhair A, et al. Radiation recall: a well recognized but neglected phenomenon. Cancer Treat Rev 2005;31(7):555–70.

Debridement Techniques and Non–Negative Pressure Wound Therapy Wound Management

Elizabeth Thompson, DVM

KEYWORDS

- Wound healing • Debridement techniques • Chronic wounds • Granulation
- Epithelialization

KEY POINTS

- The importance of initial wound classification and daily reevaluation of wound stage cannot be understated.
- Products available to enhance healing are categorized based on the stage of wound healing to which they exert their effects.
- After patient stability has been verified, thorough debridement is critical in order to create an environment conducive for healing.
- The wound environment of acute and chronic wounds differs greatly, often requiring different management approaches.

INTRODUCTION

All wound management must begin with assessing patient stability to ensure that the wound is the most imminent issue and the patient can safely undergo sedation or general anesthesia. Although some patients present in the acute stage of trauma, many cases present after a significant time lapse from initial insult, or even after numerous failed attempts at management. For this reason, the wound must be carefully evaluated and classified, because treatment recommendations differ depending on acute versus chronic nature as well as the level of contamination present. Once classified, most wounds require some degree of debridement. The presence of necrotic or foreign material, damaged tissue, and bacteria remains a nidus for infection, prolongs the inflammatory phase, and impedes wound contraction and epithelialization.[1] Once thorough debridement has been accomplished, an effort is made to stimulate

The author has nothing to disclose.
Surgery, North Carolina State University, College of Veterinary Medicine, 1060 William Moore Drive, Raleigh, NC 27606, USA
E-mail address: emthomp6@ncsu.edu

subsequent phases of healing, including production of granulation tissue, epithelialization, and wound contraction. This article aims to address wound management at each stage of wound healing, with a primary focus on various methods of debridement and products available to stimulate granulation tissue and epithelialization.

WOUND CLASSIFICATION

Initial wound evaluation begins with classification, the most common of which is a scheme developed to predict the probability that a wound will become infected. Reported risks of infection are 1% to 5% for clean wounds, 9% to 11% for clean-contaminated, 15% to 17% for contaminated, and greater than 27% for dirty wounds if they are not already infected.[1] Alternatively, the "TIME" mnemonic reported by Schultz and colleagues[2] in 2005 was developed to draw focus to specific aspects of a wound in order to more specifically identify different components of tissue damage, which may inevitably require a combined approach via various products and/or procedures to aid in healing. In this mnemonic, "T" stands for tissue (nonviable or deficient), "I" for infection/inflammation, "M" for moisture imbalance, and "E" for epidermis or edge of wound. Once the wound is classified, it can be better determined as to which treatment option will be most appropriate. First intention or primary healing is reserved for clean incisions that can be closed primarily, whereas second intention, used for contaminated or dirty wounds, requires open wound management and allows the wound to gradually close on its own via granulation tissue formation, epithelialization, and subsequent contraction. Third-intention healing, also known as delayed primary closure, involves initial open wound management until granulation tissue has developed, after which time the wound is surgically closed (**Table 1**).[3]

Wound classification must also take into account the fact that wounds present at various stages in the healing process, and identifying the current phase of wound healing will help one choose products to enhance as opposed to hinder specific phases of healing. Upon initial trauma, the inflammatory stage is initiated, leading to vasoconstriction, followed by vasodilation with increased vascular permeability to allow infiltration of the wound with cytokines, growth factors, and thromboplastin.[4] Debridement and cellular proliferation then ensue, with neutrophil infiltration occurring almost immediately, leading to oxygen-dependent killing of organisms via free radicals,[3] followed later by monocyte/macrophage infiltration, which phagocytize organisms and debris.[5] The repair phase involves connective tissue formation and wound

Table 1 Wound classifications	
Clean	Surgically induced wound with no inflammation or entrance into respiratory, alimentary, genital, or urinary tracts
Clean-contaminated	Surgically induced wound in which respiratory, alimentary, genital, or urinary tracts are entered without unusual contamination, evidence of infection, or break in sterile technique
Contaminated	Surgical wounds in which there are major breaks in sterility or gross spillage from gastrointestinal tract; incisions with acute, nonpurulent inflammation
Dirty	Old traumatic wounds, perforated viscera, or existing infection

Data from Simmons BP. CDC guideline for prevention of surgical wound infections. Infect Control 1982;3(2):187–96; and Garner JS. CDC guideline for prevention of surgical wound infections. Infect Control 1985;7(3):193–200.

contraction. The primary cells present during this phase include fibroblasts, endothelial cells, and epithelial cells. The repair phase results in angiogenesis as well as the formation of granulation tissue, which is resistant to infection and plays a role in both contraction and providing a scaffold for epithelialization. Wound maturation and remodeling finalize the healing process by strengthening newly re-formed collagen. Fibroblasts differentiate into myofibroblasts and continue to pull wound edges together, eventually leading to a scar that is about 80% original tissue strength before wounding.[3,6]

It is important to note that this pathway of wound healing is a systematic one whose stages are all required to occur in an efficient and orderly manner. If cell signaling and margination are hindered or delayed, this can lead to the formation of a chronic, non-healing wound with secondary complications.[5] Chronic wounds are characterized by dysfunctional cellular events and aberrant cytokine and growth factor activity with senescence of fibroblasts, lack of neutrophil regulation, and continued oxygen free radical production leading to chronic inflammation. Hypoxia associated with chronic wounds impairs leukocyte bactericidal action, leading to persistent proliferation of bacteria at the wound site.[7] Understanding the difference between acute and chronic wounds is important in the process of characterizing the wound because, as noted previously, requirements for healing can be significantly different.

FACTORS THAT AFFECT WOUND HEALING

There are a variety of factors that affect wound healing, and thus, a simple visual inspection and classification of the wound may not always allow one to address all confounding factors attributed to healing. Systemic factors include medications, nutrition, and systemic disease processes, such as diabetes, hyperadrenocorticism, uremia, hepatic disease, feline immunodeficiency virus, or any other disease process that impairs the immune system or negatively affects the body's ability to effectively heal.[1,8,9] Diets deficient in protein can delay wound healing, and it was found that serum protein less than 2 g/dL may delay wound strength.[10] Steroids and chemotherapy agents are common medications avoided in association with wound healing because of their impairment of the immune system. Chemotherapy drugs attack rapidly dividing cells, including fibroblast proliferation, and should be avoided whenever possible in patients with wounds.[8,9] Radiation therapy has also been noted to decrease the oxygen content in the wound to a level below that which is needed for normal wound healing, a phenomenon called fibrotic microangiopathy.[8]

Local factors include vascular supply, infection, mechanical stress, and local radiation effects. It has been shown that a microbial burden at or greater than 10^5 CFU per gram of tissue indicates infection[11]; however, other factors can predispose to infection. In 2015, Turk and colleagues[12] prospectively evaluated 846 dogs undergoing surgery in which 3% developed surgical site infections (SSI), finding that hypotension, class of surgery, and use of an implant increased the risk of SSI, and 74% of cultures revealed Staphylococcus organisms. Maintaining normothermia, normotension, normoglycemia, and appropriate tissue oxygenation have been recommended as a means of reducing the risk of SSIs.[13]

Finally, species differences are also considered primary factors affecting wound healing. The difference in cutaneous angiosomes is one primary factor, with dogs having a greater density of collateral subcutaneous trunk vessels increasing tissue perfusion and thus explaining why dogs have been shown to have improved healing properties compared with cats.[14,15] First-intention wound healing in cats was shown to have a breaking strength half of that in dogs, and second-intention healing was faster and developed more abundant granulation tissue in dogs than cats.[14] Removal of the subcutaneous tissue was also found to inhibit wound healing in both cats and dogs, although to a greater degree in cats. This factor is important in that the removal of the subcutis has been shown to reduce wound perfusion, granulation, contraction, epithelialization, and overall healing.[15,16] Knowledge of factors impacting healing is important in choosing the treatment method and products best suited for every specific wound, keeping in mind the species and localization.

DEBRIDEMENT

In a stable patient with a wound classified as contaminated or dirty, debridement is the first step in management. Debridement can be performed in a variety of ways and can be classified as selective or nonselective. Selective debridement uses endogenous or exogenous enzymes to remove only debris or damaged tissues while leaving healthy tissue intact. Nonselective debridement in the form of mechanical or hydrodynamic methods may inadvertently remove some healthy tissue along with the necrotic tissue and debris.[17] Some wounds require surgical debridement with sharp dissection to remove larger portions of necrotic or nonviable tissue, preserving questionable tissue for later removal if necessary. Once this is complete, other forms of mechanical or enzymatic debridement are often implemented to complete the debridement process in order to create an environment conducive for granulation and epithelialization (**Table 2**).

Lavage

Wound lavage is considered hydrodynamic debridement, allowing the mechanical removal of particulate matter and bacteria as well as the dilution of exudate and other toxins at the site of the wound bed. Irrigation pressures of 7 to 8 psi are recommended to remove debris and bacteria without driving microorganisms further into tissues.[18] One study found that an 18-g catheter in conjunction with a 35-cc syringe successfully obtained this pressure. In another study, however, it was found that a 1-L bag pressurized to 300 mm Hg most closely achieved 7 to 8 psi with needle gauge used being an insignificant factor.[18,19] Pressures higher than this not only allow deeper seeding of bacteria within the wound but also can cause tissue trauma and decreased resistance to infection.[20,21] Various solutions have been used for lavage, with most common recommendations including phosphate-buffered saline

Table 2	
Debridement options	
Debridement Method	**Examples**
Mechanical (selective)	• Surgical debridement
Mechanical or hydrodynamic (nonselective)	• Lavage • Wet-to-dry bandaging
Biosurgical (selective)	• Medical maggots
Autolytic (selective)	• Hydrogel • Hydrocolloid • Alginates • Polyurethane foam • Sugar • Honey • Hydrolyzed bovine collagen

or lactated Ringers, because hypotonic solutions were shown to cause destruction of canine fibroblasts.[22] Some studies have shown that tap water used to clean acute wounds was not associated with a statistically significant increase in infection when compared with saline.[23] However, when compared with phosphate-buffered solution and lactated Ringers, sterile tap water damaged canine fibroblasts at all time points, presumptively because of the alkaline pH, hypotonicity, and cytotoxic trace elements.[22] Hydrogen peroxide and sodium hypochlorite solutions have also been found to be cytotoxic to fibroblasts with resultant delay in epithelialization, and thus, in addition to tap water, cannot be recommended as wound lavage solutions.[24–26]

Chlorhexidine solution has also been evaluated for wound lavage, and studies have shown mixed results. One study indicated both 0.05% chlorhexidine diacetate and 1% povidone iodine were cytotoxic to canine fibroblasts; however, when evaluated in vivo it was found that 0.05% chlorhexidine had significantly more bactericidal activity than povidone iodine and the saline control groups, with a 6-hour residual activity level even in the presence of organic matter, and low systemic absorption and toxicity. This study suggests that concentrations of chlorhexidine diacetate that are cytotoxic to fibroblasts in vitro do not interfere with wound healing in vivo and thus may be a suitable choice for hydrodynamic debridement.[17,18,24] When looking more specifically at povidone iodine, bactericidal activity was found to be proportional to the concentration of free iodine in solution, with good efficacy against gram-positive and -negative bacteria, Candida, and fungi. It is, however, inactivated by organic matter, and thus, debridement needs to occur before lavage as opposed to using it as a source of hydrodynamic debridement.[18,24] Some studies involving povidone iodine also report complications such as acute contact dermatitis, metabolic acidosis, ototoxicity, and thyroid dysfunction, and thus, it may prove safer to use a previously listed option.[27]

Wet to dry

Wet-to-dry bandages have long been used for nonselective mechanical debridement despite a variety of reports describing their destructive nature via the removal of healthy granulation in addition to nonviable tissue and debris. The continued use of this method of debridement is largely due to the fact that it is readily available and inexpensive. It is appropriate only for mechanical debridement in the initial inflammatory and debridement phase of wound healing; thus, the wound bed should be closely evaluated after each bandage change for any evidence of granulation tissue presence, suggesting a necessary change in management protocol.[28,29]

Gauze dressing does not support optimal granulation tissue formation and wound healing. It has been shown to be more labor intensive than advanced dressings such as hydrocolloids, alginates, hydrogels, and foams.[29] In addition, gauze does not present any physical barrier to the entry of bacteria, because one study showed that bacteria traveled through 64 layers of gauze before bandage change, which can be dangerous because removal of the dried dressing disperses a significant amount of bacteria into the air.[30] Frequent wound dressings can lead to a drop in wound temperature, causing vasoconstriction and decrease in blood perfusion, also drastically impairing the ability of oxygen to clear bacteria.[30,31] Despite these various arguments, by far the most common argument against wet-to-dry bandages is the inability to maintain a moist wound environment, which has been proven to shorten wound inflammatory and proliferative phases and lead to more rapid and orderly angiogenesis, faster revascularization, and more rapid progression of wound healing.[31,32]

Maggot Therapy

The use of maggots for wound decontamination dates back to the beginnings of civilization; however, it has fallen out of favor because of patient intolerance despite documentation of efficacy, safety, and simplicity.[33] Maggot therapy is a form of both mechanical and enzymatic debridement and can be particularly useful in chronic and multidrug-infected wounds, or in patients who have significantly contaminated and necrotic tissue but have comorbidities precluding surgical debridement. The most commonly used larva, *Lucilia sericata*, produces proteolytic and antimicrobial substances as well as ammonia in the gut and salivary glands. Enzymes identified include serine, aspartyl, and metalloproteinases, which lead to liquefaction and digestion of necrotic tissues, irrigation of bacteria in the wound, as well as a change in pH, resulting in debridement, disinfection, and enhancement of the healing process.[34–36] Mechanical debridement occurs as larvae use adduction of mouth hooks to scrape and abrade necrotic tissue.[37] In vitro, maggots kill or inhibit growth of a large range of pathogenic bacteria, specifically *Staphylococcus aureus* and group A and B *Streptococcus*, as well as show activity against *Pseudomonas*. Little to no efficacy has been documented against *Escherichia coli* or *Proteus*.[38,39] Recommendations for use suggest 5 to 10 maggots per square centimeter of wound, left undisturbed for 1 to 3 days before bandage change, which involves removal with gentle irrigation.[37] In a survey of 8 veterinarians using maggot therapy in small animals, it was concluded to be safe and beneficial, avoiding amputation and euthanasia in some cases. In this study, the choice to use maggots was most commonly due to chronic wounds that had failed conventional medical or surgical therapy.[40]

MAINTAINING A MOIST WOUND ENVIRONMENT AND ENHANCING WOUND HEALING

Stages of wound healing are intertwined processes, and it may be possible to have a therapeutic agent that enhances one stage although inhibiting another, or that act to address multiple stages at once such as debridement as well as promotion of granulation tissue and epithelialization. The following products help maintain a moist environment to enhance healing processes, although several also contribute to wound debridement and minimize bacterial presence.

Hydrogel

Hydrogel occlusive dressings are composed of insoluble, hydrophilic polymers shown to enhance granulation tissue and wound contraction when compared with hydrocolloids and polyethylene occlusive dressing. When used in an occlusive dressing, these materials maintain a moist interface and prevent exudate loss from the surface of the wound, which has been shown to increase the rate of epithelialization and provide a means of painless autolytic debridement.[41–43] A unique characteristic of hydrogel is the cooling effect identified because of its high specific heat, making it capable of cooling the skin surface up to 5° and maintaining that reduced temperature for up to 6 hours, contributing to pain relief and diminution of the inflammatory response.[43] Hydrogel can also be used as a gel, paste, or composite sheet and in all forms has resulted in more rapid granulation tissue formation and wound contraction, leading to healing primarily by wound contraction, resulting in a smaller scar.[41]

Hydrocolloid

Hydrocolloids are formulations containing elastomeric, adhesive, and gelling agents that create a moist healing environment and are impermeable to moisture vapor and gasses. Their unique component is their "melting" behavior, which occurs as the dressing adsorbs exudate and forms a viscous colloidal gel that remains in the wound upon removal of the dressing.[43] They have been shown to inhibit contamination, stimulate collagen synthesis, and reduce fluid loss from wounded tissue. In a study comparing hydrocolloid and hydrogel occlusive dressings with polyethylene semiocclusive dressings, the hydrocolloid group resulted in more exuberant granulation tissue and a higher rate of positive bacterial cultures, with the residual exudate under the hydrocolloid dressing being malodorous and difficult to remove. By study end, there was significantly less total wound area healed in the hydrocolloid group. Despite data indicating that hydrogel-based products may be a better option for moist wound healing, hydrocolloid dressings remain a viable option, with specific indications (chronic wounds and burn treatment) listed in the literature.[43]

Alginates

Alginates are polysaccharide dressings derived from seaweed containing zinc and calcium with or without silver.[43] These dressings interchange the calcium in the material for sodium in the wound, forming a hydrophilic gel over the wound surface, which maintains a moist wound environment. These products are used for heavily exudative wounds, absorbing and retaining 20 to 30 times its weight in moisture.[44] The hydrophilic properties enhance granulation tissue formation and may provide hemostasis. Components of this product have been shown to bind to elastase, reducing proinflammatory cytokines and inhibiting free radicals.[45] The exudate that forms in the wound can be rinsed in between bandage changes; however, if the film created diminishes and the alginate dries, clearing it from the wound bed can damage the wound much like gauze.[43]

Porcine Small Intestinal Submucosa Dressing

Porcine small intestinal submucosa (PSIS) dressings are composed of collagen, fibronectin, hyaluronic acid, chondroitin sulfate A, heparin, heparin sulfate, and growth factors. Collagen dressings are used to enhance healing by acting as a lattice for cellular ingrowth.[46] A study of dogs with open wounds and exposed metatarsal bone evaluated the effect of PSIS on healing time, epithelialization, angiogenesis, contraction, and inflammation. There was no significant difference found in mean wound size between the control and treated groups at day 7 or day 21, although a greater mean perfusion was found in the nontreated control groups.[47] Further research is required to determine if PSIS has a place in management of open wounds.

Hydrolyzed Bovine Collagen Dressing

Hydrolyzed bovine collagen dressing promotes autolytic debridement, absorbs fluid from exudative wounds, and can act as a template or scaffold for fibroblasts to enter, resulting in newly synthesized endogenous collagen. Compared with semiocclusive nonadherent dressings, the collagen dressing was hydrophilic and enhanced the moist wound environment; however, a significant difference in epithelialization between the groups was not identified when evaluated histologically.[48] Similar to the PSIS, studies currently do not provide strong evidence for the benefit of these materials.

Polyurethane Foam

Polyurethane foam sponge dressing is a highly absorbent, permeable, nonadherent dressing primarily used in highly exudative wounds. It is classified as moisture retentive, because it absorbs excess fluid and stimulates the formation of granulation tissue. It also supports autolytic debridement, although less effectively than several other products listed.[49]

COMBATING MICROBIAL BURDEN IN WOUND CARE

Although the previously discussed management options aim to achieve more rapid wound healing, when a microbial burden is present, the benefits of these products are negated and other treatments may be necessary as an alternative or as an addition to the bandage in order to minimize bacterial load. The following products aim to achieve that goal, although there is often overlap between antimicrobial products and those that serve to debride or enhance wound healing.

Zinc

Zinc is a trace mineral that is composed of many enzymes, including DNA and RNA polymerases, and is required for protein synthesis, DNA synthesis, mitosis, and cell proliferation.[50] Studies have shown that any defect in expression of zinc transcription factors in messenger RNA coding of growth factors is consistent with impaired healing, because zinc is instrumental in stabilization of cellular membranes and closely involved in intracellular signaling and neurotransmission.[51,52] Zinc compounds have been shown to decrease/modulate the local inflammatory reaction and have been reported to have some soothing and mild analgesic effects in people via the reduction of nitric oxide (NO) formation and modulation of the local immune response.[52] These products have resulted in auto-debridement, reduction of superinfections, and enhancement of epithelialization. In a randomized controlled trial looking at effects of zinc oxide applied topically to both chronic and acute wounds, it was effective as an enzymatic topical debriding agent for healing chronic leg ulcers and proved more effective at debridement and promotion of epithelialization compared with hydrocolloid occlusive dressings.[53] Many studies involving wound healing and zinc have been conducted on chronic wounds, because the wound environment in these cases tend to have abnormal zinc metabolism and low serum zinc levels,[54] whereas studies evaluating zinc in acute wounds have failed to result in any significant improvement in healing.[55]

Silver

Elemental silver has no antibacterial action or ionic charge, unlike its cation Ag^+, which is highly reactive and toxic to multiple components of bacterial cell metabolism. Mechanisms of action include damage to bacterial cell wall, blockade of transport enzymes, alterations of proteins, and binding of DNA and RNA preventing transcription/division.[56] Silver has been incorporated into a variety of products, such as silver sulfadiazine (SSD) cream, occlusive dressings, and foam for vacuum-assisted closure. Silver demonstrates broad-spectrum antimicrobial effects on both gram-positive and -negative bacteria, including *Pseudomonas*, methicillin-resistant *S aureus*, and *Enterococcus* species.[56] Some studies indicate that silver products can retard wound contraction, although this effect may be reversed with the addition of aloe vera and nystatin.[57]

Honey

The use of honey in wounds dates back to 2000 BC and has been shown to decrease inflammatory edema, accelerate sloughing of devitalized tissue, provide a local cellular energy source, have a broad antibacterial effect, and stimulate macrophages, fibroblasts, and angiogenesis, enhancing granulation tissue and epithelialization.[58–60] In a study by Wang and colleagues,[61] it was discovered that honey combats infection via 2 independent mechanisms working in tandem: bactericidal components that actively kill cells, and also a disruption of bacterial quorum sensing, which weakens bacterial coordination and virulence. The natural glucose oxidase in honey produces gluconic acid and hydrogen peroxide from glucose, allowing an antibacterial property of peroxide, albeit at harmlessly low levels. The concentration of H_2O_2 that accumulates in 1 hour is approximately 1000 times less than that found in the H_2O_2 solution (3%) commonly used as an antiseptic. Inhibine is the antibacterial component shown to be hydrogen peroxide in the inhibine assay by the natural glucose oxidase in honey, and a direct relationship is shown between the inhibine number and the hydrogen peroxide production.[62] Honey also has a high concentration of antioxidants, helpful in protecting from free radicals that may be produced by the hydrogen peroxide.[63,64] The topical acidification of wounds has been shown to promote wound healing; therefore, honey's low pH (3.6–3.7) accelerates healing as well as increases its antibacterial effects.[65] In a 1998 study by Efem[66] comparing *Pseudomonas*-infected wounds both in vitro and in vivo, a complete inhibition of the organism did not occur on culture plates, yet all wounds containing the organism were completely sterile within 1 week of therapy, concluding that honey may have a better effect in vivo than in vitro.

Numerous varieties of honey have been tested in vitro against *S aureus*, and a highly significant difference was found in antibacterial activity with Manuka honey, maintaining its antibacterial activity in a catalase environment, indicating it also contains a nonperoxide component of activity.[61,63] Honey used to treat wounds must be unpasteurized and ideally should not be heated higher than 37°C.[60,67] There are a variety of ways honey can be applied to a wound, including but not limited to a liquid, gel, impregnated foam, or gauze, and even used as a storage medium for skin grafts.[60,68] Other major benefits for using honey include the fact that it is easily accessible and inexpensive.

Sugar

Indications for using sugar for a wound are similar to that of honey in that they have several similar effects. Sugar has been shown have rapid antibacterial action, enhances tissue formation and epithelialization, and accelerates wound healing.[69] Support for use of sugar in wound healing is based on the low water content/high osmolarity that sugar creates in a wound, which draws lymph into a wound, providing nutrition for regenerating tissues.[67] Low osmolarity also inhibits bacterial growth. Because the concentration of sugar causes migration of water and lymph out of tissues and into the sugar solution, the solution becomes diluted, and thus the activity of sugar is no longer beneficial. For this reason, large amounts of sugar must be used, and the bandage should be changed twice daily. Because of the large volume of sugar required, it has been suggested that sugar is better suited for wounds that have a defect into which it can be poured, whereas honey is better for a flatter wound surface. Individuals being treated with sugar do not develop hyperglycemia because sugar is a complex molecule and cannot be directly absorbed from the wound.[58] Once a healthy granulation bed has developed, sugar should be replaced with an alginate, hydrocolloid, or hydrogel dressing.[70]

Tripeptide Copper Complex

Tripeptide copper complex (TCC) has been shown to stimulate several biological activities in wound healing. Initially isolated from human plasma, it is described as a growth factor and chemotactic agent that increases neovascularization, epithelialization, and collagen deposition, while accelerating wound contraction.[71,72] Copper, the main component of TCC, has direct angiogenic effects by eliciting the migration of inflammatory cells as well as enhancing the mobility of the endothelium.[73] Studies have shown enhanced healing of chronic diabetic ulcers in people as well as accelerated wound healing in ischemic open wounds of rats.[74] When comparing TCC with topical zinc oxide for open wounds, those treated with TCC more rapidly developed a granulation bed and contracted more quickly, leading to expedited wound healing (Table 3).[75]

CHRONIC WOUNDS

Chronic wounds can be an entirely different entity to address, because many mechanisms that have proven effective in support of healing an acute wound may not work in a chronic environment. Alternatively, there are wound-healing products that show no major benefit in the acute wound, but aid significantly in stimulating chronic wound beds to heal. Wounds become chronic for a variety of reasons, including persistent infections, senescence of growth factors, venous stasis, systemic disease, or excessive proteolytic degradation of newly formed extracellular matrix, which, under normal circumstances, stimulate keratinocytes to proliferate and migrate.[82–86] Nonhealing wounds promote bacterial growth, inhibit penetration of antibiotics, and prevent the formation of granulation tissue and subsequent reepithelialization. The following products have specific indications in the face of chronic wounds.

Growth Factors

Growth factors and their use in chronic wound healing are a rapidly growing field of research, initially discovered by their ability to stimulate mitosis of cells in serum-free culture. Growth factors play a role in cell division, migration, differentiation, protein expression, and enzyme production.[86,87] These factors have the ability to heal wounds by stimulating angiogenesis, cell proliferation, and chemotaxis of inflammatory cells and fibroblasts. Acute wounds have many growth factors that play a crucial role in wound healing, such as platelet-derived growth factor (PDGF), but chronic wounds lose that balance.[85] The application of an autologous mixture of growth factors into the pressure ulcers has been shown to increase wound healing compared with control wounds.[88] Platelet-rich plasma (PRP) and epidermal growth factor are just a few of those used in studies looking at this promising new category of wound healing.

Platelet-Rich Plasma

PRP is a concentrated delivery of platelets that contain alpha granules that release growth factors, including PDGF, vascular endothelial growth factor, bFGF, and ILGF, among others. Proposed effects include enhanced production of collagen, proteoglycans, and fibrin matrix, as well as stimulation of angiogenesis, chemotaxis, and epithelialization. In 2014, Tambella and colleagues[89] performed a prospective, randomized, blinded, controlled clinical trial of 18 dogs with chronic bilateral wounds caused by decubital ulcers to evaluate the efficacy of autologous platelet gel treatment. They found a significantly greater mean percent reduction in wound area than nontreated wounds and a significantly faster overall healing time than wounds treated with paraffin-impregnated gauze. When comparing these results to a variety of other studies, it was noted that those looking at the use of PRP in acute wounds were unable to identify significant benefits, whereas those applying it to chronic wounds did find significant improvements in wound healing.[89,90]

Mesenchymal Stem Cells

Mesenchymal stem cells have also been used to promote chronic wound healing by increasing keratinocyte migration and proliferation, epithelialization, blood vessel production, and an increased rate of wound healing.[91,92] As normal skin depends on adult stem cells for renewal and maintenance, damaged skin, particularly chronic wounds, lack these factors. Patients at particular risk for delayed wound healing are those with bone marrow depletion, indicating a need to provide multipotent stem cells that can differentiate into those required for regeneration and healing. In 2013, Kim and colleagues[93] evaluated beagles with surgically created wounds treated with mesenchymal stem cells compared with controls. They found more rapid closure, increased collagen synthesis, cellular proliferation, and decreased expression of proinflammatory cytokines in the stem cell–treated group. They hypothesized that stem cells might exert a paracrine effect on wound healing via the promotion of fibroblast proliferation or exaggerated angiogenesis. It was also noted that at least 10^6 cells/cm^2 of tissue was required for significant therapeutic effects.[93]

Leech Therapy

Some wounds fail to heal because of vascular issues such as venous stasis. When this is the case, the use of leech therapy can be beneficial. Leeches have been used not only in wounds suffering from venous stasis but also to protect against venous congestion and to salvage replanted digits and flaps.[94–96] Leeches secrete various anticoagulant agents in their saliva, such as hirudin, bufrudin, factor Xa, and antiplatelet factors.[94] In various studies, wound healing was shown to be significantly faster after the application of leeches.[95,97] Although medicinal leeches are used in these studies, there are reports of serious infections resulting, all of which cultured positive for *Aeromonas hydrophilia* (**Table 4**).[98]

MISCELLANEOUS WOUND-HEALING THERAPIES
Low-Intensity Light Laser

Low-intensity light laser has also been evaluated to promote wound healing; however, the dose used is critical because higher intensity can create cellular damage.[101] This modality uses photoirradiation to induce cellular proliferation, collagen synthesis, growth factor release, and DNA synthesis. Other reported benefits include vasodilation and improved lymphatic drainage in addition to acceleration of angiogenesis.[101,102] A large variety exists in the literature regarding laser type and wavelength used. One guideline recommends once daily treatment for 7 to 10 days using 2 to 6 J/cm^2 for acute wounds and 2 to 8 J/cm^2 for chronic wounds.[103] A model of surgically induced wounds in diabetic rats also found that both biochemical and histopathologic parameters of wounds showed that the laser-treated group healed faster as compared with the control group.[104] Although some studies reported equivocal results in comparison to control patients, the numerous positive results make this treatment modality worthwhile for many practices willing to train hospital personnel and acquire the appropriate safety equipment, including protective eyewear for both the

Table 3
Topical wound therapies

Topical Therapy	Mechanism	Proposed Benefit	Adverse Effects Contraindications, Miscellaneous
Honey	• Natural glucose oxidase produces gluconic acid and hydrogen peroxide from glucose • Provides high concentrations of antioxidants • Disruption of bacterial quorum sensing, weakening bacterial coordination and virulence • Acidification of wounds	• Decreases inflammatory edema • Accelerates sloughing of devitalized tissue • Broad-spectrum antibacterial • Antioxidants protect from free radicals produced by hydrogen peroxide • Provides local energy source • Stimulates fibroblasts, angiogenesis • Enhances granulation tissue and epithelialization	• Recommend using unpasteurized honey • Should not be heated higher than 37°C • Manuka found to maintain better antibacterial properties compared with several other types
Sugar	• Low water content/high osmolarity, drawing lymph into the wound, providing nutrition for regenerating tissues	• Enhanced granulation tissue, epithelialization, and wound healing • Inhibits bacterial growth	• Must be used in large amounts • Quickly becomes diluted and may require more frequent bandage changes (q12h) • Should be replaced with other dressings once healthy granulation tissue is present • Not directly absorbed from the wound, thus safe in diabetic patients
Triple antibiotic ointment[76]	• Contains bacitracin zinc, neomycin sulfate, polymyxin B • Maintains moist wound environment • Noncytotoxic	• Enhanced epithelialization • Broad-spectrum antimicrobial	• Potential to delay wound contraction
Acemannan[72]	• Derived from aloe vera plant • Hydrophilic and promotes moist wound healing • Stimulates macrophages, angiogenesis, and epidermal growth	• Stimulation of angiogenesis and epithelialization	• Can exacerbate granulation tissue • May inhibit wound contraction

Agent	Mechanism	Benefits	Considerations
Maltodextrin[72]	• D-Glucose polysaccharide derived from hydrolysis of corn or potato starch • Provides a source of glucose to cells • Provides a moist wound environment • Attracts white blood cells and cytokines	• May enhance granulation tissue and provide early epithelialization	• Must flush thoroughly from wound between bandage changes
Aloe vera[77,78]	• Stimulation of fibroblast replication • Maintenance of moist wound environment • Antiprostaglandin and antithromboxane properties	• Stimulation of epithelial growth and tissue repair • Reduction of inflammation	• Due to the key role of inflammation in initial stages of wound healing, should be reserved for after inflammatory and debridement phase complete
Zinc	• Required for stabilization of cellular membranes, intracellular signaling, and neurotransmission • Modulates local inflammatory reaction and immune response • Reduces NO formation	• Auto-debridement • Antimicrobial • Enhancement of epithelialization • Analgesia	
Hydrogel	• Maintain moist environment • Painless autolytic debridement • High specific heat	• Enhance granulation tissue, epithelialization, and wound contraction • Cooling effect for pain control	
Silver/SSD cream	• Toxic to bacterial cell metabolism • Damages bacterial cell wall, blockage of transport enzymes, alteration of proteins, and binding of DNA and RNA, preventing transcription/division	• Broad-spectrum antimicrobial • Antifungal	
Chitosan[79,80]	• Derived from chitin-rich crab shell • Enhance functions of inflammatory cells and rate of inflammatory cell infiltrate into the wound bed	• Enhanced granulation tissue and epithelialization • Hemostatic agent	• May result in excess granulation tissue impaired epithelialization • Fatal hemorrhagic pneumonia reported in dogs administered 50 mg/kg subcutaneously[81]
TCC	• Copper elicits migration of inflammatory cells and enhances the mobility of endothelium	• Increases neovascularization, epithelialization, collagen deposition • Accelerated wound contraction	

Table 4
Topical stimulation for chronic wounds

Therapy	Mechanism	Proposed Benefit	Adverse Effects Contraindications, Miscellaneous
Platelet-rich plasma	• Concentrated platelets containing alpha granules, which release growth factors: PDGF, VEGF, bFGF, ILGF	• Enhanced promotion of collagen, proteoglycans, and fibrin matrix • Stimulation of angiogenesis, chemotaxis, and epithelialization	
Epidermal growth factor[99,100]	• Incorporates amino acid polypeptides, which facilitate dermal cell regeneration and migration of keratinocytes	• Enhances epithelialization	
Mesenchymal stem cells	• Increases keratinocyte migration and proliferation • Multipotent cells, which can differentiate into cells most depleted in chronic wounds	• Increases rate of epithelialization • Enhances angiogenesis • Increases collagen synthesis	• 10^6 cells/cm^2 tissue required for significant therapeutic effects
Leeches	• Secretes anticoagulant agents and antiplatelet factors	• Protective against venous stasis • Results in more rapid wound healing compared with controls	• Can cause serious wound infections due to transmission of *A hydrophilia*

staff and the patient. Potential risks associated with treatment include retinal damage, increased absorption in pigmented areas, and stimulation and alteration of cellular activity, which can be detrimental in the case of neoplastic or infected tissue. Laser treatment also leads to vasodilation, which is helpful in the wound bed but harmful over hemorrhagic tissue.[101,103]

Pulsed Electromagnetic Field

Pulsed electromagnetic field generates complex multiform pulses of oscillating electromagnetic fields in the ultralow frequency range of 0.5 to 18 Hz. The value of this therapy is based on the theory that normal tissue healing is partially mediated by endogenous bioelectric signals, and thus, this treatment modality is designed to replicate that. The anode (+) is placed on a moist sterile gauze over the wound bed while the cathode (−) is placed on the adjacent skin, so that negatively charged cells (macrophages and neutrophils) will migrate toward the anode, promoting the inflammatory stage of wound healing. Alternatively, if the cathode (−) is placed over the wound bed and the anode (+) is placed over the adjacent skin, positively charged cells (fibroblasts, keratinocytes, and epidermal cells) will migrate toward the cathode.[105] It has been shown to inhibit microbial flora and enhance wound healing in some studies; however, others have shown equivocal data, and more research is required to investigate this treatment modality.[102,106]

One form of this therapy is available in the form of a sheet incorporated into the patient's bandage. The microcurrent created by the product (JumpStart, also known as Procellera [Arthrex, Naples, FL]), uses elemental silver and zinc dot matrix on a sheet, producing a current in the range of 0.6 to 0.7 V. Kim and colleagues[107] studied the antibacterial efficacy against single-species and mixed populations of microorganisms that led to colonization and infection of wounds, finding that Jump-Start was effective against a significant number of wound pathogens. Another study found this product able to prevent biofilm formation and disrupt existing biofilm integrity via downregulation of GPDH, a necessary component of bacterial phospholipid synthesis. This study also identified silencing of quorum sensing genes and downregulation of antibiotic resistance genes.[108] There is evidence to indicate use of this product increased keratinocyte migration with more rapid epithelialization and wound healing.[109,110]

Therapeutic Ultrasound

Therapeutic ultrasound provides periodic pressure oscillations at a frequency and amplitude determined by the ultrasound source. Immediate effects are due to elevation of temperature from the absorption of sound waves. Tissues possessing higher ultrasound absorption coefficients such as bone experience higher temperature enhancements compared with muscle tissue, which possesses a lower absorption coefficient. Secondary effects, most notably cavitation, refer to rapid growth and collapse of bubbles, or sustained oscillary motion of bubbles inducing a strong physical, chemical, and biologic effect on tissues.[111] Most notable effects include enhanced tissue repair, specifically by enhancing cell proliferation and protein synthesis during the healing of skin wounds, tendons, and fractures.[112–115] Other benefits include enhanced transdermal drug delivery, reduction of antibiotic resistance of bacterial films, enhanced angiogenesis, treatment of vascular thrombosis, and enhanced periodontal wound healing and bone repair in mucoperiosteal flaps.[111,116] One source recommends ultrasonic delivery at high frequency (3 MHz) and intensity (0.1–3.0 W/cm^2) used for 5 to 10 minutes every other day, with contraindications in hemorrhagic, infected, or neoplastic tissue. Other safety concerns stem from undesired tissue interactions as well as auditory effects due to air-borne ultrasound waves. Selection of appropriate parameters is crucial for the safe use, including frequency, intensity, duty cycle, and application time.[111]

Miscellaneous wound therapies			
Therapy	Mechanism	Proposed Benefit	Adverse Effects or Contraindications
Low-intensity laser	• Photoirradiation used to induce cellular proliferation, collagen synthesis, growth factor release, and DNA synthesis	• Vasodilation, improved lymphatic drainage • Enhanced angiogenesis	• High doses can lead to cellular and tissue damage • Retinal damage • Increased absorption in pigmented areas • Contraindicated over infected, neoplastic, or hemorrhagic tissue • Once daily treatment for 7–10 d using 2–6 J/cm^2 for acute wounds and 2–8 J/cm^2 for chronic wounds

(continued on next page)

(continued)

Therapy	Mechanism	Proposed Benefit	Adverse Effects or Contraindications
Pulsed electromagnetic field	• Generates complex multiform pulses of oscillating electromagnetic fields in ultralow frequency of 0.5–18 Hz • Replicates the endogenous bioelectric signals present in normal intact tissue • Negatively charged cells (macrophages and neutrophils) migrate toward the anode • Positively charged cells (fibroblasts, keratinocytes, and epidermal cells) migrate toward the cathode • Silencing of quorum sensing genes and downregulation of antibiotic resistance genes	• Inhibits microbial flora • Enhanced granulation tissue • Prevention of biofilm formation and disruption of existing biofilm integrity	• Wound treatment recommendations indicate treatment of the wound bed for 60 min, 2–3 times daily for 5–7 d • Procellera (JumpStart) sheets provide a current of 0.6–0.7 V, must remain moist
Therapeutic ultrasound	• Induces periodic pressure oscillations, elevating the temperature of tissues due to absorption of sound waves • Leads to rapid growth and collapse of bubbles (cavitation) • Enhanced protein synthesis skin and tendon	• Enhanced transdermal drug delivery • Enhanced drug uptake in cells and tissues • Reduction of antibiotic resistance of bacterial films • Enhanced angiogenesis • Treatment of vascular thrombosis • Accelerated wound healing in periodontal tissues and bone	• Auditory impairment due to air-borne ultrasound waves • Selection of appropriate parameters critical for safe use, including frequency, intensity, duty cycle, and application time • Contraindicated in hemorrhagic, infected, or neoplastic lesions • Can interfere with pacemakers • One source recommends ultrasonic delivery at high frequency (3 MHz) and intensity (0.1–3.0 W/cm^2) used for 5–10 min every other day

SUMMARY

Ideally, wound healing should be a systematic process incorporating multiple phases in an orderly manner. For a variety of reasons, this may not always be the case, and thus, critical evaluation and classification of a wound are required before narrowing down the appropriate available treatment options. Once wound care has begun, it is equally necessary to reevaluate the wound at each bandage change, because the healing phase of the wound may have changed, requiring modifications to the treatment plan.

REFERENCES

1. Simmons BP. CDC guidelines for prevention of surgical wound infections. Infect Control 1982;3(2):187–96.
2. Schultz G, Mozingo D, Romanelli M, et al. Wound healing and TIME; new concepts and scientific applications. Wound Repair Regen 2005;13(4):S1–11.
3. Orgill D, Robert H, Demling MD. Current concepts and approaches to wound healing. Crit Care Med 1988;16(9):899–908.
4. Teller P, White TK. The physiology of wound healing: injury through maturation. Surg Clin North Am 2009;89:599–610.
5. Snyder RJ, Lantis J, Kirsner RS, et al. Macrophages: a review of their role in wound healing and their therapeutic use. Wound Repair Regen 2016;24: 613–29.
6. Dyson M. Advances in wound healing physiology: the comparative perspective. Vet Derm 1997;8:227–33.
7. Martin JM, Zenilman JM, Lazarus GS. Molecular biology: new dimensions for cutaneous biology and wound healing. J Invest Dermatol 2010;130:38–48.
8. Laing EJ. Problems in wound healing associated with chemotherapy and radiation therapy. Probl Vet Med 1990;2(3):433–41.
9. Stephens FO, Hunt TK, Jawetz E, et al. Effect of cortisone and vitamin A on wound infection. Am J Surg 1971;121(5):569–71.
10. Perez-Tamayo R, Ihnen M. The effect of methionine in experimental wound healing: a morphologic study. Am J Pathol 1953;29(2):233–49.
11. Tobin GR. Closure of contaminated wounds: biologic and technical considerations. Surg Clin North Am 1984;64(4):639–52.
12. Turk R, Singh A, Weese JS. Prospective surgical site infection surveillance in dogs. Vet Surg 2015;44:2–8.
13. Anderson DJ, Podgorny K, Berrios-Torres SI, et al. Strategies to prevent surgical site infections in acute care hospitals: 2014 update. Infect Control Hosp Epidemiol 2014;35(6):605–27.
14. Bohling MW, Henderson RA, Swaim SF, et al. Cutaneous wound healing in the cat: a macroscopic description and comparison with cutaneous wound healing in the dog. Vet Surg 2004;33:579–87.
15. Bohling MW, Henderson RA, Swaim SF, et al. Comparison of the role of subcutaneous tissues in cutaneous wound healing in the dog and cat. Vet Surg 2006; 35:3–14.
16. Fahie MA, Shettko D. Evidence-based wound management: a systematic review of therapeutic agents to enhance granulation and epithelialization. Vet Clin Small Anim 2007;37:559–77.
17. Waldron DR, Trevor P. Management of superficial skin wounds. In: Slatter DH, editor. Textbook of small animal surgery, vol. 2, 2nd edition. Philadelphia: WB Saunders; 1993. p. 269.

18. Liptak JM. An overview of topical wound management of wounds. Aust Vet J 1997;75(6):408–13.
19. Gall TT, Monnet E. Evaluation of fluid pressures of common wound-flushing techniques. Am J Vet Res 2010;71(11):1384–6.
20. Stevenson TR, Thacker JG, Rodeheaver GT, et al. Cleansing the traumatic wound by high pressure syringe irrigation. JACEP 1976;5:17–21.
21. Singer AJ, Hollander JE, Subramanian S, et al. Pressure dynamics of various irrigation techniques commonly used in the emergency department. Ann Emerg Med 1994;24:36–40.
22. Buffa EA, Lubbe AM, Verstraete FJM, et al. The effects of wound lavage solutions on canine fibroblasts: an in vitro study. Vet Surg 1997;26:460–6.
23. Fernandez R, Griffiths R. Water for wound cleansing. Cochrane Database Syst Rev 2012;(2):CD003861.
24. Swaim SF. Topical wound medications: a review. J Am Vet Med Assoc 1987;190(12):1588–93.
25. Swaim SF. Bandages and topical agents. Vet Clin North Am 1990;20(1):47–65.
26. Johnston DW. Wound healing in skin. Vet Clin North Am 1990;20(1):1–25.
27. Lozier SM. Topical wound therapy. In: Harari J, editor. Surgical complications and wound healing in small animal practice. Philidelphia: Saunders; 1993. p. 63–88.
28. Lawrence JC. Dressings and wound infection. Am J Surg 1994;167(1A):21S–4S.
29. Fleck CA. Why "wet to dry"? J Am Coll Clin Wound Spec 2009;1:109–13.
30. Lawrence JC, Lilly HA, Kidson A. Wound dressing and airborne dispersal of bacteria. Lancet 1992;339:807.
31. Wodash AJ. Wet-to-dry dressings do not provide moist wound healing. J Am Coll Clin Wound Spec 2014;4:63–6.
32. Dyson M, Young S, Pendle CL, et al. Comparison of the effects of moist and dry conditions on dermal repair. J Invest Dermatol 1988;91(5):434–9.
33. Whitaker IS, Twine C, Whitaker MJ, et al. Larval therapy from antiquity to the present days: mechanism of action, clinical applications and future potential. Postgrad Med J 2007;83:409–13.
34. Valachova I, Prochazka E, Bohova J, et al. Antibacterial properties of lucifensin in Lucilia sericata maggots after septic injury. Asian Pac J Trop Biomed 2014;4(5):358–61.
35. Valachova I, Majtan T, Takac P, et al. Identification and characterization of different proteases in Lucilia sericata medicinal maggots involved in maggot debridement therapy. J App Biomed 2014;12:171–7.
36. White SH, Wimley WC, Selsted ME. Structure, function, and membrane integration of defensins. Curr Opin Struct Biol 1995;5:521–7.
37. Jones G, Wall R. Maggot therapy in veterinary medicine. Res Vet Sci 2008;85(2):394–8.
38. Kerridge A, Lappin-Scott H, Stevens JR. Antibacterial properties of larval secretions of the blowfly, Lucilia sericata. Med Vet Entomol 2005;19:333–7.
39. Bonn D. Maggot therapy: an alternative for wound infection. Lancet 2000;356:1174.
40. Sherman RA, Stevens H, Ng D, et al. Treating wounds in small animals with maggot debridement therapy: a survey of practitioners. Vet J 2007;173:138–43.
41. Morgan PW, Binnington AG, Miller CW, et al. The effect of occlusive and semi-occlusive dressings on the healing of acute full-thickness skin wounds on the forelimbs of dogs. Vet Surg 1994;23:494–502.

42. Bolton LL, Johnson CL, Van Rijswijk L, et al. Occlusive dressings: therapeutic agents and effects on drug delivery. Clin Dermatol 1991;9(4):573–83.

43. Helfman T, Ovington L, Falanga V. Occlusive dressings and wound healing. Clin Dermatol 1994;12:121–7.

44. Zbigniew A, Wojciech B. Burn wounds management with occlusive dressings granuflex 1B in dogs. In: WSAVA Conference Proceedings. 2002. Available at: http://www.vin.com/apputil/content/defaultadv1.aspx?pId=11147&id=3846403. Accessed November 1, 2016.

45. Wiegand C, Heinze T, Hipler UC. Comparative in vitro study on cytotoxicity, antimicrobial activity, and binding capacity for pathophysiological factors in chronic wounds of alginate and silver-containing alginate. Wound Repair Regen 2009; 17(4):511–21.

46. Swaim SF. Wound management offers new alternatives. DVM Best Practices 2002;4–6.

47. Winkler JT, Swaim SF, Sartin EA, et al. The effect of porcine-derived small intestinal submucosa product on wounds with exposed bone in dogs. Vet Surg 2002; 31:541–51.

48. Swaim SF, Gillette RL, Sartin EA, et al. Effects of a hydrolyzed collagen dressing on the healing of open wounds in dogs. Am J Vet Res 2000;61(12):1574–8.

49. Banks V, Bale S, Harding K, et al. Evaluation of a new polyurethane foam dressing. J Wound Care 1997;6(6):266–9.

50. Andrews M, Gallagher-Allred C. The role of zinc in wound healing. Adv Wound Care 1999;12:137–8.

51. Scrimshaw NS, Young VR. The requirements of human nutrition. Sci Am 1976; 235:50–64.

52. Lansdown AB, Mirastschijski U, Stubbs N, et al. Zinc in wound healing: theoretical, experimental, and clinical aspects. Wound Repair Regen 2007;15:2–16.

53. Agren MS, Ostenfeld U, Kallehave F, et al. A randomized, double blind, placebo controlled multicenter trial evaluating topical zinc oxide for acute open wounds following pilonidal disease excision. Wound Repair Regen 2006;14:526–35.

54. Henzel JH, DeWeese MS, Lichti EL. Zinc concentrations within healing wounds. Significance of postoperative zincuria on availability and requirements during tissue repair. Arch Surg 1970;100:349–57.

55. Kaufman KL, Mann FA, Kim DY, et al. Evaluation of the effects of topical zinc gluconate in wound healing. Vet Surg 2014;43(8):972–82.

56. Leaper DJ. Silver dressings: their role in wound management. Int Wound J 2006; 3:282–94.

57. Muller MJ, Hollyoak MA, Moaveni Z, et al. Retardation of wound healing by silver sulfadiazine is reversed by aloe vera and nystatin. Burns 2003;29(8):834–6.

58. Kamat N. Use of sugar in infected wounds. Trop Doct 1995;23(4):185.

59. Molan PC. The role of honey in the management of wounds. J Wound Care 1999;8(8):415–8.

60. Mathews KA, Binnington AG. Wound management using honey. Compendium 2002;24(1):52–60.

61. Wang R, Starkey M, Hazan R, et al. Honey's ability to counter bacterial infection arises from both bactericidal compounds and QS inhibition. Front Microb 2012; 144(3):1–8.

62. White JW, Subers MH, Schepartz AI. The identification of inhibine, the antibacterial factor in honey, as hydrogen peroxide and its origin in a honey glucose-oxidase system. Biochem Biophys Acta 1963;73:57–70.

63. Hyslop PA, Hinshaw DB, Scraufstatter IU, et al. Hydrogen peroxide as a potent bacteriostatic antibiotic: implications for host defense. Free Radic Biol Med 1995;19(1):31–7.

64. Kwakman PH, Van de Akker JP, Guclu A, et al. Medical grade honey kills antibiotic resistant bacteria in vitro and eradicates skin colonization. Clin Infect Dis 2008;46(11):1677–82.

65. Kaufman T, Eichenlaub EH, Angel MF. Topical acidification promotes healing of experimental deep partial thickness skin burns: a randomized double-blind preliminary study. Burns Incl Therm Inj 1985;12:84–90.

66. Efem SEE. Clinical observations on the wound healing properties of honey. Br J Surg 1998;75:679–81.

67. Molan PC, Cooper RA. Honey and sugar as a dressing for wounds and ulcers. Trop Doct 2000;30:249–51.

68. O'Connell K, Wardlaw JL. Unique therapies for difficult wounds. Today's Vet Pract 2011;1(1):10–6.

69. Mathews KA, Binnington AG. Wound management using sugar. Compendium 2002;24(1):41–50.

70. Dawson J. The role of sugar in wound healing: a comparative trial of the healing of infected wounds using traditional gauze/antiseptic packing, and granulated sugar. Ann R Coll Surg Engl 1996;78(2):82–5.

71. Swaim SF, Bradley DM, spano JS, et al. Evaluation of multipeptide-copper complex medications on open wound healing in dogs. J Am Anim Hosp Assoc 1993; 29:519–25.

72. Swaim S, Gillette R. An update on wound medications and dressings. Compendium 1998;20:1133–44.

73. Raju KS, Alessandri G, Ziche M, et al. Ceruloplasmin, copper ions, and angiogenesis. J Natl Cancer Inst 1982;69:1183–8.

74. Mulder GD, Patt LM, Sanders L, et al. Enhanced healing of ulcers in patients with diabetes by topical treatment of glycyl-l-histidyl-l-lysine copper. Wound Repair Regen 1994;2:256–69.

75. Canapp SO, Farese JP, Schultz GS, et al. The effect of topical tripeptide-copper complex on healing of ischemic open wounds. Vet Surg 2003;32:515–23.

76. Lee AH, Swaim SF, Yang ST, et al. Effects of gentamicin solution and cream on the healing of open wounds. Am J Vet Res 1984;45(8):1487–92.

77. Rodriguez-Bigas M, Cruz NI, Suarez A. Comparative evaluation of aloe vera in the management of burn wounds in guinea pigs. Plast Reconstr Surg 1988;81: 386–9.

78. Swaim SF, Riddell KP, McGuire JA. Effects of topical medications on the healing of open pad wounds in dogs. J Am Anim Hosp Assoc 1992;28:499–502.

79. Ueno H, Mori T, Fujinaga T. Topical formulations and wound healing applications of chitosan. Adv Drug Deliv Rev 2001;52(2):105–15.

80. Okamoto Y, Shibazaki K, Miniama S, et al. Evaluation of chitin and chitosan on open wound healing in dogs. J Vet Med Sci 1995;57(5):851–4.

81. Shigemasa Y, Minami S. Applications of chitin and chitosan for biomaterials. Biotechnol Genet Eng Rev 1996;13:383–420.

82. Cook H, Davies KJ, Harding KG, et al. Defective extracellular matrix reorganization by chronic wound fibroblasts is associated with alterations in the TIMP-1, TIMP-2, and MMP-2 activity. J Invest Dermatol 2000;115:225–33.

83. Hasan A, Murata H, Falabella A, et al. Dermal fibroblasts from venous ulcers are unresponsive to action of transforming growth factor beta 1. J Dermatol Sci 1997;16:59–66.

84. Schultz GS, Barillo DJ, Mozingo DW, et al. Wound bed preparation and a brief history of TIME. Int Wound J 2004;1:19–31.
85. Stadelmann WK, Digenis AG, Tobin GR. Physiology and healing dynamics of chronic cutaneous wounds. Am J Surg 1998;176(2A):26S–38S.
86. Bennett NT, Schultz GS. Growth factors and wound healing: biochemical properties of growth factors and their receptors. Am J Surg 1993;165:729–37.
87. Bennett NT, Shultz GS. Growth factors and wound healing: part II. Role in normal and chronic wound healing. Am J Surg 1993;166:74–81.
88. Knightin DR, Fiegel VD, Austin LL, et al. Classifications and treatment of chronic non-healing wounds. Ann Surg 1986;204:322–30.
89. Tambella AM, Attili AR, Dini F, et al. Autologous platelet gel to treat chronic decubital ulcers: a randomized, blind controlled clinical trial in dogs. Vet Surg 2014;43:726–33.
90. Karayannopoulou M, Psalla D, Kazakos G, et al. Effect of locally injected autologous platelet-rich plasma on second intention wound healing of acute full-thickness skin defects in dogs. Vet Comp Orthop Traumatol 2015;3:172–8.
91. Falanga V, Iwamoto S, Chartier M, et al. Autologous bone marrow-derived vulture mesenchymal stem cells delivered in a fibrin spray accelerate healing in murine and human cutaneous wounds. Tissue Eng 2007;13(6):1299–312.
92. Chen L, Tredget EE, Wu PYG, et al. Paracrine factors of mesenchymal stem cells recruit macrophages and endothelial lineage cells and enhance wound healing. PLoS One 2008;3(4):1–12.
93. Kim JW, Lee JH, Lyoo YS, et al. The effects of topical mesenchymal stem cell transplantation in canine experimental cutaneous wounds. Vet Derm 2013;24:242–53.
94. Abdualkader AM, Ghawi AM, Alaama M, et al. Leech therapeutic applications. Ind J Pharm Sci 2013;75:127–37.
95. Grobe A, Michalsen A, Hanken H, et al. Leech therapy in reconstructive maxillofacial surgery. J Oral Maxillofac Surg 2012;70:221–7.
96. Weinfeld AB, Yuksel E, Boutros S, et al. Clinical and scientific considerations in leech therapy for the management of acute venous congestion: an updated review. Ann Plast Surg 2000;45:207–12.
97. Darestani KD, Mirghazanfari SM, Moghaddam KG, et al. Leech therapy for linear incisional skin wound healing in rats. J Acupunct Meridian Stud 2014;7(4):194–201.
98. Schnabl SM, Kunz C, Unglaub F, et al. Acute postoperative infection with Aeromonas hydrophilia after using medical leeches for treatment of venous congestion. Arch Orthop Trauma Surg 2010;130(10):1323–8.
99. Tanaka A, Nagate T, Matsuda H. Acceleration of wound healing by gelatin film dressings in epidermal growth factor. J Vet Med Sci 2005;67(9):909–13.
100. Eisinger M, Sadan S, Soehnchen R, et al. Wound healing by epidermal derived factors: experimental and preliminary clinical studies. Prog Clin Biol Res 1988;266:291–302.
101. Kloth LC. Electrical stimulation for wound healing: a review of evidence from in vitro studies, animal experiments, and clinical trials. Int J Low Extrem Wounds 2005;4:23–44.
102. Lucroy MD, Edwards BJ, Madewell BR. Low-intensity laser light-induced closure of a chronic wound in a dog. Vet Surg 1999;57(5):851–4.
103. Millis DL, Saunders DG. Laser therapy in canine rehabilitation. In: Millis DL, Levine D, editors. Canine rehabilitation and physical therapy. 2nd edition. Philadelphia: Elsevier; 2014. p. 359–80.

104. Maiya GA, Kumar P, Rao L. Effect of low intensity helium-neon (He-Ne) laser irradiation on diabetic wound healing dynamics. Photomed Laser Surg 2005;23(2): 187–90.

105. Belanger AY. Therapeutic electrophysical agents: evidence behind practice. 2nd edition. Philadelphia: Lippincott Williams & Wikins; 2013.

106. Scardino MS, Swaim SF, Sartin EA, et al. Evaluation of treatment with a pulsed electromagnetic field on wound healing, clinicopathologic variables, and central nervous system activity of dogs. Am J Vet Res 1998;59(9):1177–81.

107. Kim H, Makin I, Skiba J, et al. Antibacterial efficacy testing of a bioelectric wound dressing against clinical wound pathogens. Open Microbiol J 2014;8: 15–21.

108. Banerjee J, Ghatak PD, Roy S, et al. Improvement of human keratinocyte migration by a redox active bioelectric dressing. PLoS One 2014;9(3):1–14.

109. Whitcomb E, Monroe N, Hope-Higman J, et al. Demonstration of a microcurrent-generating wound care device for wound healing within a rehabilitation center patient population. J Am Coll Clin Wound Spec 2012;4(2):32–9.

110. Blount AL, Foster S, Rapp DA, et al. The use of bioelectric dressing in skin graft harvest sites: a prospective case series. J Burn Care Res 2012;33(3):354–7.

111. Mitragotri S. Healing sound: The use of ultrasound in drug delivery and other therapeutic applications. Nat Rev Drug Discov 2005;4(3):256–60.

112. Freitas TP, Gomes M, Fraga DB, et al. Effect of therapeutic pulsed ultrasound on lipoperoxidation and fibrogenesis in an animal model of wound healing. J Surg Res 2010;161(1):168–71.

113. Webster DF, Harvey W, Dyson M. The role of ultrasound-induced cavitation in the "in vitro" stimulation of collagen synthesis in human fibroblasts. Ultrasonics 1980;18:33.

114. Enwemeka CS, Rodriquez O, Mendosa S. The biomechanical effects of low-intensity ultrasound on healing tendons. Ultrasound Med Biol 1990;16:801.

115. Duarte LR. The stimulation of bone growth by ultrasound. Arch Orthop Trauma Surg 1983;101:153.

116. Tamura IH, Watanabe T, Itou M. Low-intensity pulsed ultrasound accelerates periodontal wound healing after flap surgery. J Periodontal Res 2008;43:212–6.

Negative Pressure Wound Therapy

Bryden J. Stanley, BVMS, MACVSc, MVetSc

KEYWORDS

- Negative pressure wound therapy • Dressings • Healing • Skin • Wound

KEY POINTS

- Negative pressure wound therapy (NPWT) transforms an open wound into a closed, moist environment through which a controlled vacuum is applied.
- The modality is widely used in human medicine in acute, subacute, and chronic open wounds; plastic and reconstructive surgery; dehiscences; open abdominal drainage; and closed incisions.
- NPWT has been shown to reduce interstitial edema, stimulate fibroplasia, and enhance angiogenesis, although some mechanisms remain to be elucidated.
- Veterinary studies have recently shown that NPWT is beneficial in open wounds, in which it promotes the early appearance of a smooth granulation tissue bed; NPWT also improves free graft survival and has been used in several other indications.
- Further studies are needed to refine NPWT protocols for different species, to identify different indications, and to determine which protocols are best suited for each application type.

 Video content accompanies this article at http://www.vetsmall.theclinics.com.

INTRODUCTION TO NEGATIVE PRESSURE WOUND THERAPY

Open wounds are regularly addressed in veterinary medicine and can be challenging to manage, especially when there is significant loss of full-thickness skin (**Fig. 1**). Injuries include traumatic anatomic degloving wounds, shear injuries, penetrations, avulsions resulting in physiologic degloving, envenomations, burns, necrotizing fasciitis or vasculitides, incisional dehiscences, and surgical wounds left open to heal by second intention. Involvement of the underlying subdermal fat, fascia, muscle, and even bone may compromise perfusion and impede healing of the tissues. Traumatic wounds are typically contaminated or infected and additionally may contain devitalized tissues and foreign debris. Management of these wounds is intensive, requiring repeated debridement and lavage events. Multiple dressing changes over a prolonged

Disclosure: The author has nothing to disclose.
College of Veterinary Medicine, Michigan State University, 736 Wilson Road, East Lansing, MI 48824, USA
E-mail address: stanle32@cvm.msu.edu

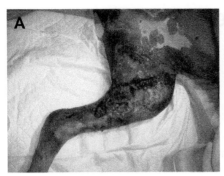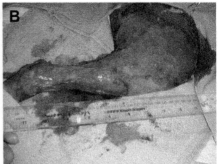

Fig. 1. Significant loss of full-thickness skin from a variety of causes is a frequent presentation in small animal medicine. (*A*) A 3-year-old spayed female boxer with physiologic degloving to medial left pelvic limb. (*B*) The same wound following cleansing, lavage, and debridement.

period have traditionally been necessary, often continuing through the inflammatory phase into the proliferative phase of healing. Intensive wound care continues until the wound is either suitable for a reconstructive procedure or until it has largely healed by second intention and can be managed in the home setting.

During the early phase of wound healing, dressings have historically been changed frequently with saline-dampened wet-to-dry dressings to aid in ongoing debridement and exudate management.[1] Although effective in the inflammatory phase, these bandage changes require daily sedation, and significant nursing time and expenditure on consumables. As the understanding of the cellular and molecular events orchestrating wound healing increased in the last half-century, the importance of the extracellular matrix was appreciated.[2–6] Subsequently, many modern wound dressings and biologics have been developed, not just to protect but also to nurture the wound, resulting in an extensive choice of products. Several mechanical adjuncts have also been developed to enhance wound healing over the last few decades, including electromagnetic stimulation, magnetic therapy, ultrasonography therapy, radiofrequency energy, low-intensity laser, hydrosurgical debridement, oxygen therapies, and negative pressure wound therapy (NPWT).[7–11] Of these, NPWT has shown particular clinical advantages, not only for open wound management but also in reconstructive, orthopedic, and general surgical applications.[12–17]

NPWT refers to the application of a vacuum evenly distributed across the surface of a wound, typically through a foam dressing. An open-cell polyurethane or polyvinyl alcohol foam is conformed to the wound and sealed from the environment with occlusive drapes. Specialized access tubing connects the dressing to a programmable vacuum pump, which subjects the entire wound to an evenly distributed negative pressure. Wound exudate is collected in a canister attached to the pump (**Fig. 2**). The level of vacuum is programmable, ranging from 75 to 150 mm Hg with 125 mm Hg being commonly used for open wounds.[18] NPWT can be continuously, cyclically, or intermittently applied.[19] There are several synonymous terminologies for NPWT, including topical negative pressure therapy, vacuum-assisted closure, subatmospheric wound therapy, closed-suction wound drainage, and microdeformational wound therapy.[20–24]

MECHANISMS OF ACTION

The aims of the NPWT modality are to remove wound exudate; decrease interstitial edema; draw wound edges together; promote blood supply to the wound; and, by

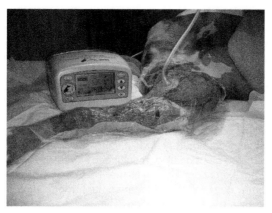

Fig. 2. The same dog as in **Fig. 1**, with NPWT applied to the wound. An open-cell polyure-thane foam has been conformed to the wound and sealed from the environment with occlusive drapes. Tubing connects the dressing to a programmable vacuum pump and wound exudate is collected in a canister attached to the pump.

applying mechanical strain, stimulate cells involved with modulating the inflammatory and proliferative response to injury.[19]

Early studies to investigate the effects of NPWT on full-thickness wounds were performed in swine. These studies concluded that, at −125 mm Hg, NPWT increases blood flow to a wound, accelerates the rate of granulation tissue formation, decreases bacterial counts, and improves flap survival.[25,26] Despite a lack of mechanistic proof, the modality rapidly penetrated human wound care and trauma departments, largely because of its remarkable clinical outcomes.[27–32] NPWT was subsequently adopted into other surgical applications, such as free skin grafts, pedicled muscle and skin flaps, incisional dehiscences, cytotoxic sloughs, complex orthopedic trauma, envenomations, extravasations, and burns.[33–36] There is no doubt that NPWT has revolutionized wound management. It is the modality of choice to address complex soft tissue wounds sustained in the US military.[37,38] More recently, it has been used for abdominal drainage and incisional management.[13–15]

Although new therapeutic applications for NPWT continue to be reported, the physiologic, cellular, and molecular mechanisms of the modality are still being elucidated.[19,39] Animal and human clinical studies support the original data showing that chronic, subacute, and acute wounds, flaps, and free grafts respond favorably to NPWT.[20,40–42] The originally reported increase in wound perfusion was corroborated, although an area of hypoperfusion adjacent to the wound edge that rebounded following termination of NPWT was also reported.[43,44] An earlier appearance of granulation tissue was also substantiated, with intermittent or variable NPWT shown to be more effective at stimulating fibroplasia and neovascularization than continuous mode.[45–48] It is postulated that the benefits result from the cycling of increased blood flow (facilitating oxygenation and nutrient supply) and decreased blood flow (hypoxic stimulation of angiogenesis and fibroplasia). The evidence regarding the role of NPWT in bacterial clearance remains conflicting, with some studies showing no difference or an increase in bacterial load, despite the positive effect on wound healing.[49–52]

It is also postulated, and some data show, that the strain and microdeformation induced by NPWT on the cells within the wound, and the creation of a hypoxic gradient within the microenvironment, promotes cell recruitment, proliferation, and differentiation, resulting in enhanced neovascularization and fibroplasia.[22,53,54] The mechanical strain of negative pressure on fibroblasts seems to stimulate them to divide and increase collagen synthesis through mechanotransduction.[54–56] The mechanical deformation of other cells within and around the wound and shear forces that deform the extracellular matrix are also thought to result in a higher mitotic rate and increased production of granulation tissue.

To facilitate understanding of the underlying molecular mechanism of how NPWT enhances wound healing, a systematic review of studies that had evaluated the effects of NPWT on cytokine and growth factor expression profiles was performed.[57] This review concluded that the promotion of wound healing with NPWT occurs by modulation of cytokines to an antiinflammatory profile, and mechanoreceptor-mediated and chemoreceptor-mediated cell signaling, resulting in angiogenesis, extracellular matrix remodeling, and deposition of granulation tissue. The mechanism of enhanced wound healing is likely from a combination of local immune modulation, mechanoreceptor stimulation, and hypoxia-mediated signaling.[57]

NEGATIVE PRESSURE WOUND THERAPY IN VETERINARY MEDICINE

Experience with NPWT in veterinary medicine is not as extensive as in human medicine; the literature consists of a few controlled studies, several case series, some reviews, and many case reports in a variety of species, including dogs, cats, horses, a tiger, a tortoise, and a rhinoceros.[58–82] NPWT has also been reported successfully in avians.[83] Results have been promising for many indications in veterinary medicine, including acute open wounds, dehiscences, burns, skin grafts, skin flaps, pad transfers, perforating thoracic trauma, high-risk incisions, and open abdomens. It is likely that this modality will be widely adopted for companion animals, becoming an invaluable adjunct to wound management and other surgical applications in both large and small animals.

One of the earliest veterinary reports was a clinical case series evaluating outcomes in 15 dogs with traumatic extremity open wounds.[59] Following NPWT, all animals experienced rapid appearance of granulation tissue within the wounds and underwent successful reconstruction at an average of 4.6 days (range, 2–7 days). Complications were considered minor and included dermatitis at the wound margin and loss of vacuum causing wound desiccation. Subsequently, a randomized, controlled, experimental study in dogs compared NPWT with standard-of-care wound management in 20 forelimb wounds on 10 dogs.[64] Granulation tissue appeared in the NPWT wounds significantly earlier (day 2) than in the control wounds (day 7), and the granulating bed was smoother in the NPWT wounds than in the control wounds (**Fig. 3**). However, the NPWT wounds did not contract or epithelialize as well as the control wounds after days 7 and 11 respectively. On histology, NPWT wounds appeared to reach an acute inflammation peak earlier than control wounds, transitioning into the proliferative phase more rapidly. The modality has been shown to be well tolerated and allows several days between dressing changes in the inflammatory phase, in which previously daily bandage changes were indicated. It is often used to shorten the time period to surgical closure but can also be used into the proliferative phase.[81] Time to healing in dogs when NPWT is used is significantly shortened compared with both nonadhesive impregnated gauze dressings and highly absorbent foam dressings.[72] Overall, these studies show that NPWT is a valuable mechanical adjunct to healing in large, complicated wounds, providing a bridge to reconstruction. In addition to the enhanced wound healing effects of NPWT, the distinct logistical advantage of the prolonged time between dressing changes (up to 72 hours) compares favorably with the traditional daily wet-to-dry dressing for open wounds still in the inflammatory phase.

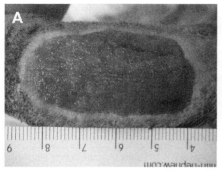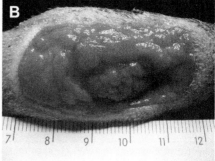

Fig. 3. (*A*) This 14-day wound in a dog has received NPWT. (*B*) This 14-day wound received a wet-to-dry dressing for 48 hours, then a Telfa dressing. Note how the granulation tissue is smoother in the wound under NPWT.

Several studies have additionally shown the feasibility and beneficial effects of NPWT in securing and enhancing acceptance of free full-thickness skin grafting in dogs and cats.[59,66,76,77,82] Not only does granulation tissue appear earlier in the interstices of the meshed graft but the open meshes close more rapidly, and percentage of graft take is higher. There is also better early adhesion of the graft to the recipient bed when under NPWT, and decreased reported seroma formation. It seems that NPWT can be used to optimize graft survival, and it may be especially valuable for large grafting procedures in which immobilization is challenging.

NPWT has also been reported as being used successfully over high-risk skin flaps and closed incisions.[61,68,73,78,80] These reports support the use of NPWT over incisions that are at high risk of complications such as swelling, infection, dehiscence caused by tension or motion, and necrosis, but further studies are indicated.

There are more than 14 different commercially available NPWT systems on the market, several of which have penetrated the veterinary market.[19,84] Some of the more advanced modifications associated with NPWT, such as concurrent instillation therapy and abdominal sepsis management, have also been reported in veterinary patients.[62,63,74] Ad hoc negative pressure devices have been devised in resource-poor settings, in both human and veterinary hospitals. These devices tend to use moistened wide-weave gauze or sterile speaker foam with negative pressure generated by hospital suction pumps.[85] The efficacy of these systems compared with commercial systems has not been rigorously evaluated.

NPWT shows much promise to enhance veterinary wound care and reconstruction and commercial veterinary units are now used throughout referral institutions in North America, Europe, and the United Kingdom. Although most NPWT is used in hospital patients, smaller mobile units can be used in the home setting. It can be used in the hospital setting as well as in the home in selected cases. However, as in human wound care, further controlled studies are indicated, not only to further the understanding of the mechanisms of the modality but also for optimizing the methodology. Given the widespread use of NPWT in human and veterinary medicine, it is important to develop robust guidelines and protocols for different indications.[85]

INDICATIONS/CONTRAINDICATIONS OF NEGATIVE PRESSURE WOUND THERAPY

Early treatment of contaminated or dirty wounds is intended to provide an environment conducive to healing by removing devitalized tissue and debris, decreasing the bacterial bioburden, preventing further contamination, and providing effective

Table 1
Wound indications for negative pressure wound therapy

Type of Wound	Description	Comments
Acute, subacute, traumatic	Including anatomic degloving and shear wounds with exposed bone	NPWT dressing is placed following cleansing, debridement, and lavage
Acute surgical wounds, managed open	Useful in preparing wound bed for grafting, also if significant contamination occurred intraoperatively	NPWT dressing is placed while patient is still in the operating room
Physiologic degloving	Cutaneous blood supply is disrupted from underlying fascia	Fenestrate the skin in several areas, and place NPWT dressing over the affected area
Necrotizing fasciitis or vasculitis	Necrotizing lesions of unknown cause. Early establishment of extent of compromise is recommended before NPWT	NPWT dressing is placed following cleansing, debridement, and lavage. Wound should be checked in 24–48 h
Abscesses	Large deep abscesses associated with edema	NPWT dressing is placed following lancing and lavage
Burn	Superficial or full thickness	NPWT can be applied with silver-impregnated dressing
Chronic wounds	Including decubital ulcers and atypical infections. Address underlying cause concurrently (eg, relieve pressure, microbial work-up, search for foreign body)	NPWT can stimulate a chronic wound to a proliferative phase
Multiple wounds	Bite wounds or stab wounds	Several wounds can be connected by connecting strips of foam between the NPWT dressings
Dehisced incisions, sloughs	Including over exposed orthopedic implants	NPWT dressing is placed following cleansing, debridement, and lavage. Shortens time to revisional closure
Skin flaps	Large flaps in mobile areas	NPWT decreases seroma and edema formation
Skin grafts	Mesh the graft generously	NPWT increases survival and immobilizes the graft-bed interface. Use moistened polyvinyl alcohol foam
Closed surgical incisions	High-risk incisions: under tension, when swelling is expected; eg, arthrodeses	NPWT decreases seroma and edema formation
Myofascial compartment syndrome	Rare indication but reported	NPWT dressing is placed following fasciotomy

Data from Refs.[12,33,61,64,69,73,75,80–82,84,89]

Box 1
Contraindications for negative pressure wound therapy
Poor periwound skin condition
Necrotic or clearly devitalized tissue
Coagulopathy
Exposed major blood vessels
Open joint
Neoplastic malignancy in the wound
Unexplored draining tract
Untreated osteomyelitis
Small wounds
Lack of overnight care

drainage.[86] There are established, incontrovertible principles of wound management that have been well proven in injuries sustained over centuries of warfare.[87,88] These principles involve thorough cleansing of the periwound and wound, debridement of necrotic and devitalized tissues, and copious pressured lavage. These main tenets of open wound management should never be neglected, regardless of the dressing that is placed on the wound. Highly exudative, traumatic wounds are ideal for NPWT. The clinical applications and indications for NPWT in small animals have been discussed and are outlined in **Table 1**.[81,84,89] There are certain wound conditions that are not suited for NPWT in veterinary medicine (**Box 1**). Before managing a wound, assess the patient's overall cardiovascular, respiratory, and neurologic status, look for comorbid conditions, and administer an appropriate level of analgesia.

TECHNIQUE
Preparation Tips

- Be meticulous on initial application of the NPWT dressing. Careful initial preparation to ensure the integrity of the seal on the periwound saves time and frustration later.

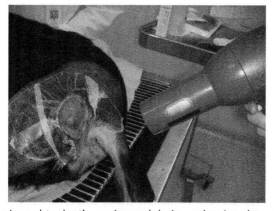

Fig. 4. A hairdryer is used to dry the periwound during a dressing change.

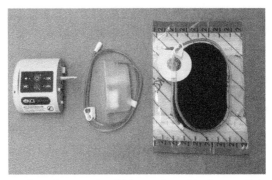

Fig. 5. All the required equipment should be gathered before applying NPWT dressings. This equipment includes, from left to right, the vacuum pump, the tubing and canister, the foam dressing, adhesive drapes, and specialized pad with tubing.

- The NPWT dressing should be applied to a wound that has already been clipped, cleansed, debrided, and lavaged. The periwound skin should be clipped and prepped with margins of 3 to 5 cm, to ensure adequate contact area for the adhesive drape. The last cleanse of the periwound skin should be with alcohol, which is an effective defatting and drying agent.
- Ensure the periwound skin is completely dry, because any moisture weakens adhesion of the drape. A hairdryer on a low setting can be used (**Fig. 4**).
- Note that the foam must be porous (open-cell or reticulated), with every air pocket communicating. Closed-cell foam mattress material is contraindicated; it does not apply an effective vacuum to the wound surface and simply becomes an occlusive dressing, leading to wound maceration.
- NPWT is typically applied to the wound when the animal is under general anesthesia, although reapplication can often be undertaken with just sedation. Aseptic technique should be maintained throughout the dressing application.
- There is a learning curve associated with this modality. Once the team becomes adept at placing the dressing and managing the vacuum pump controls, complications with dressing leakage or pump alarms will decrease.

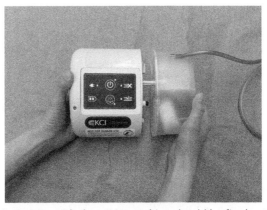

Fig. 6. The reservoir canister with the canister tubing should be firmly attached to the vacuum pump.

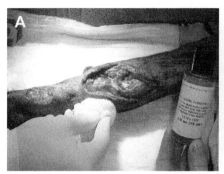
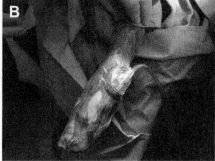

Fig. 7. (*A*) Liquid skin adhesive is applied sparingly to the periwound skin. (*B*) In areas where the periwound skin is uneven, such as in between the digits of this dog, stoma paste or hydrocolloid gels can be molded to help attain an airtight seal.

Application of Negative Pressure Wound Therapy

1. Ensure that the battery of the NPWT machine is charged and that all required equipment is gathered together (**Fig. 5**).
2. Place the reservoir canister with the canister tubing onto the vacuum pump (**Fig. 6**).
3. Check again that the skin around the wound is closely shaved or clipped, and absolutely dry. Any oozing of blood or wound fluid onto the periwound skin should immediately be swabbed from the skin with sterile gauze. Apply a thin coating of liquid skin adhesive to the skin for about 3 to 5 cm around the wound, allowing it to dry for a few minutes. If there are uneven surfaces, such as between the digits or in skin folds, stoma paste or hydrocolloid gels can be molded into a dam to help secure an airtight seal (**Fig. 7**).
4. Cut the foam dressing to the shape of the wound and place it into the wound bed. The dressing should fit just inside the wound edge to avoid compression of the wound edge and adjacent periwound skin. If the wound is large and/or irregular, the foam dressing can be roughly secured to the wound edge with a few skin staples or cut strips of adhesive drape to prevent dislodgement while the adhesive drape is applied (**Fig. 8**).

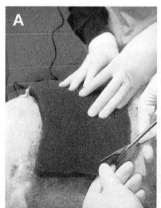
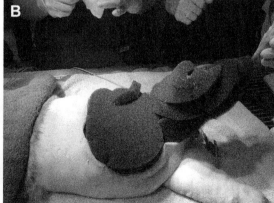

Fig. 8. (*A*) The foam is being cut to the shape of the open wound. (*B*) In larger, complex wounds the foam can be preventing from dislodging by stapling to the skin edges.

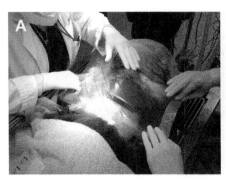
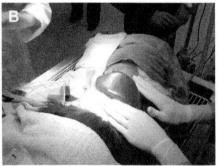

Fig. 9. (*A, B*) The wound and foam are sealed by applying the adhesive drapes and peeling off the layers as instructed. Try to avoid wrinkles in the drapes.

5. Seal the whole wound area with the impermeable, adhesive drapes. These drapes typically come sandwiched between 2 layers to facilitate handling and placement. Avoid wrinkles or folds in the drape when possible, because they can track air from the environment and compromise the integrity of the dressing (**Fig. 9**).
6. Cut a 2-cm round hole in the sheet exposing a small area of the foam dressing. Place the proprietary adhesive fenestrated disc with associated evacuation tubing over the hole (**Fig. 10**).
7. Immediately connect the evacuation tubing to the tubing on the reservoir canister of the programmable vacuum pump and set either continuous or intermittent negative pressure to the sealed wound, between −80 and −125 mm Hg. Once powered on, the dressing should contract noticeably, become very firm and raisinlike to the touch (**Fig. 11**, Video 1). As the pump approaches the preset vacuum level, it becomes quiet and only activates on an intermittent basis, to maintain the vacuum. Listen closely to the dressing for sounds of leakage (a low, moist, whistling sound); more adhesive draping may be required.
8. If the wound is on a limb, the NPWT dressing can be covered with a soft, padded bandage, coiling a length of the evacuation tubing into the bandage layers. It is useful to create a window in the bandage so that the foam dressing can be palpated, and to obtain confirmation that it is still firm and raisinlike (**Fig. 12**). With trunk wounds, the dressing can be left unbandaged. Allow adequate tubing to extend from the bandage to the patient's dorsum throughout a full range of motion if the

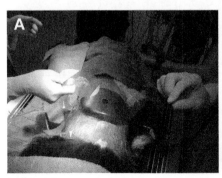
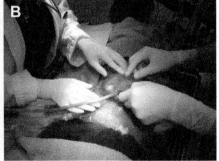

Fig. 10. (*A*) A 2-cm hole has been cut in the drape, exposing the foam. (*B*) The specialized adhesive pad with the evacuation tubing is placed over the hole.

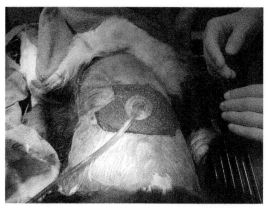

Fig. 11. NPWT has been activated and the foam dressing shrinks and becomes firm to the touch.

patient is ambulatory. However, do not allow too much slack so that the patient could become tangled. With large dogs, the pump can be inserted into a vest and worn; with small dogs and cats, it should reside immediately outside the cage, and be transported with the dog when ambulating (**Fig. 13**).

9. Dressing integrity and machine function should be checked regularly during the period of deployment. The animal should be either continually monitored in an intensive care unit or checked every 2 hours. If the vacuum is lost for more than several hours, the dressing will become occlusive and wound maceration will result.

MANAGEMENT AND COMPLICATIONS

- NPWT is redressed every 48 to 72 hours; an acute traumatic wound typically requires only 1 to 3 dressing changes before a healthy bed of granulation tissue is

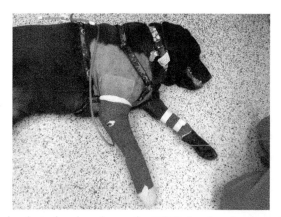

Fig. 12. The limb has been bandaged over the NPWT dressing, incorporating a coil of the evacuation tubing within its layers. A window has been cut in this bandage over the NPWT dressing. This window allows the carer to check that the dressing is still contracted down and firm to the touch.

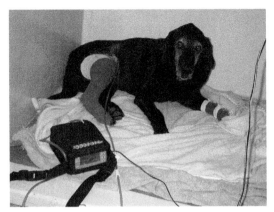

Fig. 13. Many pumps come with their own carrying satchel to facilitate ambulating with the patient.

evident. It is important not to leave the dressing on for longer than 72 hours, especially in young dogs, because granulation tissue can develop quickly and may grow into the interstices of the foam.

- Dressing changes take approximately 15 minutes and are usually performed under sedation or brief anesthesia. The entire dressing and adhesive drapes can be removed or just the portion of the dressing over the wound. In the latter case, the drape at the foam edge is sharply incised and just the foam and drape covering the foam are removed. Following wound cleansing, and placement of the new foam dressing, the adhesive drapes are placed over foam and also cover the original drapes on the periwound skin (**Fig. 14**).

- Pumps are designed to alarm with loss of pressure caused by disruption of the occlusive dressing. In this case, either reinforce the dressing with more adhesive drapes or change the dressing as soon as possible (within 2–4 hours) to prevent wound maceration. To prevent leakage of the dressing, be meticulous during original dressing placement.

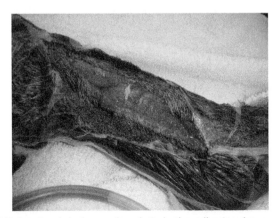

Fig. 14. The NPWT dressing is being replaced. Only the adhesive drape over the foam has been removed. Following cleansing, new foam will be placed in the wound and the adhesive drape placed, covering the original adhesive drape.

- Pumps are also designed to alarm when obstructed. This problem does not occur often because of the low viscosity of wound exudate in companion animals, and the regular venting of the tubing in some commercial systems. Obstruction can also be cleared by flushing and stripping the tubing.
- Intermittent therapy (5 minutes on, 2 minutes off) may lead to an increased risk of loss of dressing integrity caused by the lack of vacuum in the off mode. Dogs tolerate both intermittent and continuous therapy modes well, but cats sometimes seem to resent the restarting of the vacuum in intermittent mode.[81] For these reasons, NPWT is mostly used in continuous mode.

SUMMARY

NPWT is increasingly playing a beneficial role in wound care, and the modality has now been validated in several applications in veterinary medicine. Advantages of NPWT include early appearance and improved quality of granulation tissue, decreased frequency of dressing changes, elimination of strike-through (because all exudate is collected in the canister), and an earlier time to reconstruction. Further investigations are indicated to determine optimal protocols for the different indications and in different species.

SUPPLEMENTARY DATA

Supplementary data related to this article can be found online at http://dx.doi.org/10.1016/j.cvsm.2017.06.006.

REFERENCES

1. Manring MM, Hawk A, Calhoun JH, et al. Treatment of war wounds: a historical review. Clin Orthop Relat Res 2009;467(8):2168–91.
2. Schultz GS, Wysocki A. Interactions between extracellular matrix and growth factors in wound healing. Wound Repair Regen 2009;17(2):153–62.
3. Barrientos S, Stojadinovic O, Golinko MS, et al. Growth factors and cytokines in wound healing. Wound Repair Regen 2008;16(5):585–601.
4. Winter GD, Scales JT. Effect of air drying and dressings on the surface of a wound. Nature 1963;197:91–2.
5. Winter GD. Effect of air exposure and occlusion on experimental human skin wounds. Nature 1963;200:378–9.
6. Stanley BJ, Cornell K. Wound healing. In: Johnston SA, Tobias KM, editors. Veterinary surgery small animal, vol. 1, 2nd edition. St Louis (MO): Elsevier; 2018. p. 132–48.
7. Ennis WJ, Lee C, Gellada K, et al. Advanced technologies to improve wound healing: electrical stimulation, vibration therapy, and ultrasound–what is the evidence? Plast Reconstr Surg 2016;138(3 Suppl):94S–104S.
8. Friedman HI, Fitzmaurice M, Lefaivre JF, et al. An evidence-based appraisal of the use of hyperbaric oxygen on flaps and grafts. Plast Reconstr Surg 2006;117(7 Suppl):175S–90S [discussion: 191S–2S].
9. Kurach LM, Stanley BJ, Gazzola KM, et al. The effect of low-level laser therapy on the healing of open wounds in dogs. Vet Surg 2015;44(8):988–96.
10. Apelqvist J, Willy C, Fagerdahl AM, et al. EWMA document: negative pressure wound therapy. J Wound Care 2017;26(Sup3):S1–154.

11. Chen B, Kao HK, Dong Z, et al. Complementary effects of negative-pressure wound therapy and pulsed radiofrequency energy on cutaneous wound healing in diabetic mice. Plast Reconstr Surg 2017;139(1):105–17.

12. Guy H, Grothier L. Using negative pressure therapy in wound healing. Nurs Times 2012;108(36):16, 18, 20.

13. Willy C, Agarwal A, Andersen CA, et al. Closed incision negative pressure therapy: international multidisciplinary consensus recommendations. Int Wound J 2017;14(2):385–98.

14. Seternes A, Rekstad LC, Mo S, et al. Open abdomen treated with negative pressure wound therapy: indications, management and survival. World J Surg 2017; 41(1):152–61.

15. Bobkiewicz A, Walczak D, Smolinski S, et al. Management of enteroatmospheric fistula with negative pressure wound therapy in open abdomen treatment: a multicentre observational study. Int Wound J 2017;14(1):255–64.

16. Dedmond BT, Kortesis B, Punger K, et al. The use of negative-pressure wound therapy (NPWT) in the temporary treatment of soft-tissue injuries associated with high-energy open tibial shaft fractures. J Orthop Trauma 2007;21(1):11–7.

17. Argenta LC, Morykwas MJ, Marks MW, et al. Vacuum-assisted closure: state of clinic art. Plast Reconstr Surg 2006;117(7 Suppl):127S–42S.

18. Peinemann F, Sauerland S. Negative-pressure wound therapy: systematic review of randomized controlled trials. Dtsch Arztebl Int 2011;108(22):381–9.

19. Glass GE, Nanchahal J. The methodology of negative pressure wound therapy: separating fact from fiction. J Plast Reconstr Aesthet Surg 2012;65(8):989–1001.

20. Argenta LC, Morykwas MJ. Vacuum-assisted closure: a new method for wound control and treatment: clinical experience. Ann Plast Surg 1997;38(6):563–76 [discussion: 577].

21. Dorafshar AH, Franczyk M, Gottlieb LJ, et al. A prospective randomized trial comparing subatmospheric wound therapy with a sealed gauze dressing and the standard vacuum-assisted closure device. Ann Plast Surg 2012;69(1):79–84.

22. Erba P, Ogawa R, Ackermann M, et al. Angiogenesis in wounds treated by microdeformational wound therapy. Ann Surg 2011;253(2):402–9.

23. Huang C, Leavitt T, Bayer LR, et al. Effect of negative pressure wound therapy on wound healing. Curr Probl Surg 2014;51(7):301–31.

24. Orgill DP, Bayer LR. Negative pressure wound therapy: past, present and future. Int Wound J 2013;10(Suppl 1):15–9.

25. Morykwas MJ, Argenta LC, Shelton-Brown EI, et al. Vacuum-assisted closure: a new method for wound control and treatment: animal studies and basic foundation. Ann Plast Surg 1997;38(6):553–62.

26. Morykwas MJ, Faler BJ, Pearce DJ, et al. Effects of varying levels of subatmospheric pressure on the rate of granulation tissue formation in experimental wounds in swine. Ann Plast Surg 2001;47(5):547–51.

27. Mendonca DA. Negative pressure wound therapy: an important adjunct to wound care. South Med J 2006;99(6):562–3.

28. Mendonca DA, Papini R, Price PE. Negative-pressure wound therapy: a snapshot of the evidence. Int Wound J 2006;3(4):261–71.

29. Hunter JE, Teot L, Horch R, et al. Evidence-based medicine: vacuum-assisted closure in wound care management. Int Wound J 2007;4(3):256–69.

30. Kanakaris NK, Thanasas C, Keramaris N, et al. The efficacy of negative pressure wound therapy in the management of lower extremity trauma: review of clinical evidence. Injury 2007;38(Suppl 5):S9–18.

31. Gregor S, Maegele M, Sauerland S, et al. Negative pressure wound therapy: a vacuum of evidence? Arch Surg 2008;143(2):189–96.
32. Moues CM, Heule F, Hovius SE. A review of topical negative pressure therapy in wound healing: sufficient evidence? Am J Surg 2011;201(4):544–56.
33. Banwell PE, Musgrave M. Topical negative pressure therapy: mechanisms and indications. Int Wound J 2004;1(2):95–106.
34. Banwell PE. Topical negative pressure wound therapy: advances in burn wound management. Ostomy Wound Manage 2004;50(11A Suppl):9S–14S.
35. Venturi ML, Attinger CE, Mesbahi AN, et al. Mechanisms and clinical applications of the vacuum-assisted closure (VAC) device: a review. Am J Clin Dermatol 2005; 6(3):185–94.
36. Llanos S, Danilla S, Barraza C, et al. Effectiveness of negative pressure closure in the integration of split thickness skin grafts: a randomized, double-masked, controlled trial. Ann Surg 2006;244(5):700–5.
37. Geiger S, McCormick F, Chou R, et al. War wounds: lessons learned from Operation Iraqi Freedom. Plast Reconstr Surg 2008;122(1):146–53.
38. Couch KS, Stojadinovic A. Negative-pressure wound therapy in the military: lessons learned. Plast Reconstr Surg 2011;127(Suppl 1):117S–30S.
39. Lalezari S, Lee CJ, Borovikova AA, et al. Deconstructing negative pressure wound therapy. Int Wound J 2017;14(4):649–57.
40. Blackburn JH 2nd, Boemi L, Hall WW, et al. Negative-pressure dressings as a bolster for skin grafts. Ann Plast Surg 1998;40(5):453–7.
41. Schneider AM, Morykwas MJ, Argenta LC. A new and reliable method of securing skin grafts to the difficult recipient bed. Plast Reconstr Surg 1998;102(4):1195–8.
42. Chang KP, Tsai CC, Lin TM, et al. An alternative dressing for skin graft immobilization: negative pressure dressing. Burns 2001;27(8):839–42.
43. Chen SZ, Li J, Li XY, et al. Effects of vacuum-assisted closure on wound microcirculation: an experimental study. Asian J Surg 2005;28(3):211–7.
44. Wackenfors A, Sjogren J, Gustafsson R, et al. Effects of vacuum-assisted closure therapy on inguinal wound edge microvascular blood flow. Wound Repair Regen 2004;12(6):600–6.
45. Malmsjo M, Gustafsson L, Lindstedt S, et al. The effects of variable, intermittent, and continuous negative pressure wound therapy, using foam or gauze, on wound contraction, granulation tissue formation, and ingrowth into the wound filler. Eplasty 2012;12:e5.
46. Borgquist O, Gustafsson L, Ingemansson R, et al. Micro- and macromechanical effects on the wound bed of negative pressure wound therapy using gauze and foam. Ann Plast Surg 2010;64(6):789–93.
47. Borgquist O, Ingemansson R, Malmsjo M. The effect of intermittent and variable negative pressure wound therapy on wound edge microvascular blood flow. Ostomy Wound Manage 2010;56(3):60–7.
48. Borgquist O, Ingemansson R, Malmsjo M. Wound edge microvascular blood flow during negative-pressure wound therapy: examining the effects of pressures from -10 to -175 mmHg. Plast Reconstr Surg 2010;125(2):502–9.
49. Braakenburg A, Obdeijn MC, Feitz R, et al. The clinical efficacy and cost effectiveness of the vacuum-assisted closure technique in the management of acute and chronic wounds: a randomized controlled trial. Plast Reconstr Surg 2006; 118(2):390–7 [discussion: 398–400].
50. Moues CM, Vos MC, van den Bemd GJ, et al. Bacterial load in relation to vacuum-assisted closure wound therapy: a prospective randomized trial. Wound Repair Regen 2004;12(1):11–7.

51. Morykwas MJ, Simpson J, Punger K, et al. Vacuum-assisted closure: state of basic research and physiologic foundation. Plast Reconstr Surg 2006;117(7 Suppl):121S–6S.

52. Patmo AS, Krijnen P, Tuinebreijer WE, et al. The effect of vacuum-assisted closure on the bacterial load and type of bacteria: a systematic review. Adv Wound Care (New Rochelle) 2014;3(5):383–9.

53. Pietramaggiori G, Liu P, Scherer SS, et al. Tensile forces stimulate vascular remodeling and epidermal cell proliferation in living skin. Ann Surg 2007;246(5): 896–902.

54. Saxena V, Hwang CW, Huang S, et al. Vacuum-assisted closure: microdeformations of wounds and cell proliferation. Plast Reconstr Surg 2004;114(5): 1086–96 [discussion 1097–8].

55. Nishimura K, Blume P, Ohgi S, et al. Effect of different frequencies of tensile strain on human dermal fibroblast proliferation and survival. Wound Repair Regen 2007; 15(5):646–56.

56. Jacobs S, Simhaee DA, Marsano A, et al. Efficacy and mechanisms of vacuum-assisted closure (VAC) therapy in promoting wound healing: a rodent model. J Plast Reconstr Aesthet Surg 2009;62(10):1331–8.

57. Glass GE, Murphy GF, Esmaeili A, et al. Systematic review of molecular mechanism of action of negative-pressure wound therapy. Br J Surg 2014;101(13): 1627–36.

58. Adkesson MJ, Travis EK, Weber MA, et al. Vacuum-assisted closure for treatment of a deep shell abscess and osteomyelitis in a tortoise. J Am Vet Med Assoc 2007;231(8):1249–54.

59. Ben-Amotz R, Lanz OI, Miller JM, et al. The use of vacuum-assisted closure therapy for the treatment of distal extremity wounds in 15 dogs. Vet Surg 2007;36(7): 684–90.

60. Bertran J, Farrell M, Fitzpatrick N. Successful wound healing over exposed metal implants using vacuum-assisted wound closure in a dog. J Small Anim Pract 2013;54(7):381–5.

61. Bristow PC, Perry KL, Halfacree ZJ, et al. Use of vacuum-assisted closure to maintain viability of a skin flap in a dog. J Am Vet Med Assoc 2013;243(6):863–8.

62. Buote NJ, Havig ME. The use of vacuum-assisted closure in the management of septic peritonitis in six dogs. J Am Anim Hosp Assoc 2012;48(3):164–71.

63. Cioffi KM, Schmiedt CW, Cornell KK, et al. Retrospective evaluation of vacuum-assisted peritoneal drainage for the treatment of septic peritonitis in dogs and cats: 8 cases (2003-2010). J Vet Emerg Crit Care (San Antonio) 2012;22(5): 601–9.

64. Demaria M, Stanley BJ, Hauptman JG, et al. Effects of negative pressure wound therapy on healing of open wounds in dogs. Vet Surg 2011;40(6):658–69.

65. Gemeinhardt KD, Molnar JA. Vacuum-assisted closure for management of a traumatic neck wound in a horse. Equine Vet Educ 2005;17(1):27–33.

66. Guille AE, Tseng LW, Orsher RJ. Use of vacuum-assisted closure for management of a large skin wound in a cat. J Am Vet Med Assoc 2007;230(11):1669–73.

67. Harrison TM, Stanley BJ, Sikarskie JG, et al. Surgical amputation of a digit and vacuum-assisted-closure (V.A.C.) management in a case of osteomyelitis and wound care in an eastern black rhinoceros (Diceros bicornis michaeli). J Zoo Wildl Med 2011;42(2):317–21.

68. Lafortune M, Fleming GJ, Wheeler JL, et al. Wound management in a juvenile tiger (Panthera tigris) with vacuum-assisted closure (V.A.C. Therapy). J Zoo Wildl Med 2007;38(2):341–4.

69. Mullally C, Carey K, Seshadri R. Use of a nanocrystalline silver dressing and vacuum-assisted closure in a severely burned dog. J Vet Emerg Crit Care (San Antonio) 2010;20(4):456–63.

70. Nolff MC, Fehr M, Reese S, et al. Retrospective comparison of negative-pressure wound therapy and silver-coated foam dressings in open-wound treatment in cats. J Feline Med Surg 2017;19(6):624–30.

71. Nolff MC, Pieper K, Meyer-Lindenberg A. Treatment of a perforating thoracic bite wound in a dog with negative pressure wound therapy. J Am Vet Med Assoc 2016;249(7):794–800.

72. Nolff MC, Fehr M, Bolling A, et al. Negative pressure wound therapy, silver coated foam dressing and conventional bandages in open wound treatment in dogs. A retrospective comparison of 50 paired cases. Vet Comp Orthop Traumatol 2015; 28(1):30–8.

73. Nolff MC, Flatz KM, Meyer-Lindenberg A. Preventive incisional negative pressure wound therapy (Prevena) for an at-risk-surgical closure in a female Rottweiler. Schweiz Arch Tierheilkd 2015;157(2):105–9.

74. Nolff MC, Layer A, Meyer-Lindenberg A. Negative pressure wound therapy with instillation for body wall reconstruction using an artificial mesh in a Dachshund. Aust Vet J 2015;93(10):367–72.

75. Nolff MC, Meyer-Lindenberg A. Necrotising fasciitis in a domestic shorthair cat–negative pressure wound therapy assisted debridement and reconstruction. J Small Anim Pract 2015;56(4):281–4.

76. Nolff MC, Meyer-Lindenberg A. Negative pressure wound therapy augmented full-thickness free skin grafting in the cat: outcome in 10 grafts transferred to six cats. J Feline Med Surg 2015;17(12):1041–8.

77. Or M, Van Goethem B, Kitshoff A, et al. Negative pressure wound therapy using polyvinyl alcohol foam to bolster full-thickness mesh skin grafts in dogs. Vet Surg 2017;46(3):389–95.

78. Or M, Van Goethem B, Polis I, et al. Pedicle digital pad transfer and negative pressure wound therapy for reconstruction of the weight-bearing surface after complete digital loss in a dog. Vet Comp Orthop Traumatol 2015;28(2):140–4.

79. Owen LJ, Hotston Moore A, Holt PE. Vacuum-assisted wound closure following urine-induced skin and thigh muscle necrosis in a cat. Vet Comp Orthop Traumatol 2009;22:417–21.

80. Perry KL, Rutherford L, Sajik DM, et al. A preliminary study of the effect of closed incision management with negative pressure wound therapy over high-risk incisions. BMC Vet Res 2015;11:279.

81. Pitt KA, Stanley BJ. Negative pressure wound therapy: experience in 45 dogs. Vet Surg 2014;43(4):380–7.

82. Stanley BJ, Pitt KA, Weder CD, et al. Effects of negative pressure wound therapy on healing of free full-thickness skin grafts in dogs. Vet Surg 2013;42(5):511–22.

83. Knapp-Hoch H, de Matis R. Clinical technique: negative pressure wound therapy - general principles and use in avian species. Journal of Exotic Pet Medicine 2014;23:56–66.

84. Nolff MC, Meyer-Lindenberg A. Negative pressure wound therapy (NPWT) in small animal medicine. Mechanisms of action, applications and indications. Tierarztl Prax Ausg K Kleintiere Heimtiere 2016;44(1):26–37 [quiz: 38; in German].

85. Newton K, Wordworth M, Allan AY, et al. Negative pressure wound therapy for traumatic wounds. Cochrane database of systematic reviews 2017;1. Available at: http://onlinelibrary.wiley.com/doi/10.1002/14651858.CD012522/full.

86. Pavletic MM. Wound management principles and techniques. Vet Q 1997; 19(sup1):22–4.
87. Broughton G 2nd, Janis JE, Attinger CE. A brief history of wound care. Plast Reconstr Surg 2006;117(7 Suppl):6S–11S.
88. Shepard GH, Rich NM. Treatment of the soft tissue war wound by the American military surgeon: a historical resume. Mil Med 1972;137(7):264–6.
89. Kirkby KA, Wheeler JL, Farese JP, et al. Surgical views: vacuum-assisted wound closure: clinical applications. Compend Contin Educ Vet 2010;32(3):E1–6 [quiz: E7].

Wound Closure, Tension-Relieving Techniques, and Local Flaps

Laura C. Cuddy, MVB, MS[a,b],*

KEYWORDS

- Wound closure • Tension • Local flap • Subdermal plexus

KEY POINTS

- The simplest method of wound closure that is deemed to have the highest chance of success should be chosen.
- Simple tension-relieving techniques, such as undermining, strong subcutaneous sutures and walking sutures, are effective in facilitating primary wound closure in many cases.
- More advanced methods of relieving wound tension include the use of releasing incisions, skin stretchers, and tissue expanders.
- Local flaps are elevated adjacent to the recipient bed and rely on the subdermal plexus for their blood supply.
- The risk of necrosis of local flaps can be minimized with meticulous surgical technique; various modalities may be used to salvage a failing flap.

INTRODUCTION

Closure of traumatic wounds or planned surgical incisions is commonly performed in small animals. The use of local skin to cover a defect by direct apposition of the skin edges reduces the time and care otherwise required for a wound to heal by contraction and epithelialization. With direct apposition of the skin edges, cutaneous healing can proceed directly by reepithelialization.[1] The skin of dogs and cats is viscoelastic and present in abundance, meaning many wounds can be closed by adhering to basic surgical principles. The goal should be to obtain rapid wound closure using the simplest technique associated with the lowest morbidity and cost. Although the simplest technique should be chosen, this should not be at the expense of probable

Disclosure Statement: The author has nothing to disclose.
[a] Vets Now 24/7 Emergency and Specialty Hospital, 98 Bury Old Road, Whitefield, Manchester M45 6TQ, UK; [b] Veterinary Specialists, Clonmahon, Summerhill, County Meath A83 KR62, Ireland
* Veterinary Specialists, Clonmahon, Summerhill, County Meath A83 KR62, Ireland.
E-mail address: laura.cuddy@vetspecialists.ie

success because choosing an inappropriate technique will lead to more cost in the long term. A "reconstructive ladder" has been adapted for veterinary use to assist with decision making in wound closure.[2]

Before wound closure, the wound bed should be free of contamination and infection and have an adequate blood supply. If a wound is planned, for example a mass excision, then steps may be taken preoperatively to ensure there is adequate skin available for wound closure. Surgeons should have a reasonable knowledge of reconstructive techniques and multiple plans in mind when embarking on wound closure, because not every eventuality can be predicted preoperatively. Every effort should be taken to minimize wound tension; if tension is present on the wound edges, then dehiscence is likely to occur. Tension-relieving techniques act to reduce or redistribute tension from the skin edges. Recruiting neighboring skin in the form of local flaps is useful for more challenging defects where primary skin closure is not otherwise possible.

CATEGORIES OF WOUND CLOSURE
Primary Wound Closure (First-Intention Healing)

Primary closure is the immediate closure of viable tissue without tension, typically by suturing.[1] The decision as to whether a wound may be closed primarily depends on wound factors (time from wounding, manner in which wound was created, location, size, degree of contamination, availability of local tissue) and systemic factors (concurrent disease, age, malnutrition).[1,3] In healthy patients, wounds less than 3 to 6 hours old with no visible devitalized tissue or debris after lavage are candidates for primary closure; if a wound contains more than 10^5 bacteria per gram of tissue, the risk of infection is markedly increased.[1,4] Clean and clean contaminated wounds are eligible for primary closure; some contaminated wounds that can be converted to clean wounds by debridement and lavage may also be considered.[4] Dirty or infected wounds may be closed primarily only if they are first completely excised.

Where possible, wounds should be closed in a linear or curvilinear fashion because wound dehiscence is most likely to occur where incisions intersect (T, X, or Y).[5] Many wounds can be converted into fusiform defects to facilitate this closure.[6] Wounds should be sutured accurately and atraumatically with swaged on fine suture material.[2] Using a toothed Adson tissue forceps to manipulate the skin provides a firm grip that requires less pressure and inflicts less crushing injury than the Adson-Brown tissue forceps, although both have been described as more traumatic than the DeBakey thumb forceps.[6,7] Suture material should be chosen that approximates the normal strength of the tissue and loses its tensile strength concomitant to the rate of recovery of wound strength.[1] It is important to obliterate dead space; however, the number of sutures and suture size (and therefore total amount of suture material) should be kept to a minimum.[4] Skin closure may be completed using intradermal or cutaneous sutures, skin staples, or tissue adhesives.[1] Skin sutures should be placed 3 to 5 mm from wound edges to avoid increased collagenases near the wound edge, and 5 mm apart.[2] The use of reverse cutting needles decreases the risk of skin sutures cutting out through the skin edge; the depth of suture bites can be adjusted to precisely appose the wound edges and avoid step defects. In the short term, increased swelling or erythema may be seen with intradermal patterns due to increased tissue handling.[8]

If there is a small discrepancy between the length of the apposing skin edges, "fudging" is a simple technique to minimize the development of dog-ears; tissue bites are taken closer together on the shorter skin edge and further apart on the longer skin edge.[1,3] Suturing by the rule of halves is another useful technique. The wound edges are first apposed with towel clamps, and then an interrupted deep subcutaneous suture is placed at the center of the wound. Interrupted deep subcutaneous sutures are subsequently placed to continuously halve the remaining defects.[6]

Dog-ears may occur at the ends of various shaped defects, if the long axis of a fusiform incision is too short, if there is significant length discrepancy between apposing skin edges, or following movement of skin flaps into position. Dog-ears can be removed at the time of surgery but otherwise tend to remodel over several months.

There are several methods described to correct dog-ears[9]:

1. Extend the original incision through the dog-ear and excise the resulting 2 triangles of skin.
2. Incise the dog-ear along one side of its base and remove the resulting large triangle of skin. This will result in a slightly curved end to the incision.
3. Extend the fusiform incision.
4. Remove an arrowhead-shaped section of skin from the dog-ear and close the resultant "Y"-shaped incision.
5. Make a right-angle incision at end of wound and remove the excess skin to create an "L"-shaped closure.
6. Pass a suture through the upper half of the skin and tie to flatten a small dog-ear.

Delayed Primary Wound Closure

Delayed primary closure is performed 3 to 5 days after wounding, before the appearance of granulation tissue.[4] In the interim, open wound management is performed to optimize health of the wound bed before closure. This technique is used for clean contaminated or contaminated wounds where tissue viability may be questionable, or in the face of tension.[4]

Secondary Wound Closure (Third-Intention Healing)

Secondary wound closure is performed over 5 days after injury, after the appearance of a granulation bed. Secondary wound closure is typically used for contaminated or dirty wounds.[4] Excessive granulation tissue and epithelialized skin edges are debrided before wound closure.

Second-Intention Healing

Second-intention healing is where wounds are allowed to heal by granulation, contraction, and epithelialization. Permitting a wound to heal by second intention should be considered if the wound is not suitable for other techniques, in large defects, or if a significant amount of tissue is devitalized.[4] This method of healing is more protracted and often results in a less cosmetic and more fragile scar.

TENSION-RELIEVING TECHNIQUES

The cardinal rule of wound closure is to avoid tension on the skin edges. If wound edges are apposed under tension, the wound will likely go on to dehisce. Judging the amount of tension that will be tolerated is more an art than a science; it has been described that the subjective evaluation of tension is the most important decision made in wound care.[10] The properties of skin (inherent elasticity, stress relaxation, mechanical creep) in dogs and cats lend themselves to tension-relieving techniques to facilitate primary wound closure. Tension can be reduced in each layer by performing a 3-layer closure where possible: deep subcutaneous, subcutaneous, and skin.[1]

General Points

Tension lines

Tension lines, or Langer lines in humans, were first characterized in dogs in 1966.[11] The orientation of these skin tension lines reflects the predominant pull of the collagen and elastin fibers in underlying dermal and hypodermal tissues.[3] Where possible, closure should be performed parallel to tension lines; wounds closed perpendicular to tension lines are subject to greater tension, are harder to close, and carry a greater risk of wound dehiscence.[3] Tension line orientation is less critical in a patient with an abundance of skin, for example, a Bassett hound. Although knowledge of tension lines is helpful, when deciding the direction of creation or closure of a specific wound, it is more helpful to manually grasp, elevate, and push the adjacent skin to assess its availability.

Patient positioning

Careful attention should be paid to how the patient is positioned for wound closure. The patient's own body weight or tension on tied limbs may be restricting access to otherwise usable skin. Conversely, if tension is overly artificially decreased during wound closure, excessive tension may be noted when the patient is awake and weight-bearing, and this may require revision.[1]

Basic Techniques

Undermining

Undermining is most straightforward technique to mobilize skin during primary wound closure. The skin edge is elevated using minimally traumatic thumb forceps or skin hooks and is separated from the underlying tissue using a Metzenbaum scissors. The plane of dissection is in the loose areolar tissue below the dermis; if a panniculus carnosus muscle layer is present, the skin should be undermined below it in order to preserve the subdermal plexus and direct cutaneous vessels.[12] A combination of blunt and sharp dissection is used; in areas with loose areolar hypodermal tissue, scissors should be inserted into that plane with the blades closed and withdrawn with them open, whereas dense fascial attachments may be cut sharply.[3] Care should be taken to preserve any direct cutaneous vessels that are encountered. It has been described that the skin on either side of the defect should be undermined for a distance at least equal to the width of the defect; more practically undermining should be performed until the wound edges approximate without excessive tension.[6,9]

Strong subcutaneous sutures

A good subcutaneous closure should result in the skin edges being almost apposed and under no tension. Bites of the subcutaneous tissues should be taken in the fibrous portion of the hypodermis rather than in fatty tissue.[10,13] Using Backhaus towel clamps to temporarily approximate the skin edges can facilitate placement of several interrupted subcutaneous sutures, followed by a continuous subcutaneous pattern and fine skin sutures to adjust the epidermis.[10] Monofilament absorbable suture material swaged on to a 3/8 or 1/2 circle, taper or tapercut needle is most appropriate[1]; the knot should be tied at the deep part of the suture loop to prevent it from later exteriorizing.[10]

Effect of skin closures

The conclusions of a recent biomechanical study evaluating 4 different skin closure techniques infer that external skin sutures may be preferable to internal for the closure of incisions that are under tension.[14] When subjected to biomechanical distraction, interrupted and cruciate patterns withstood higher tension and maintained skin apposition better than continuous intradermal and subdermal patterns.[14] Tissue adhesives are not recommended for use in tissues under tension, even in combination with minimal nylon sutures, because they demonstrate a marked decrease in wound strength.[15] Skin staples are not recommended for use in wound edges that are under moderate tension.[1]

Walking sutures

Walking sutures were first described by Swaim[16] in 1976 as a means to move skin across a defect, obliterate dead space, and evenly distribute tension further away from the wound edges. Walking sutures mobilize skin from the periphery either toward the center or toward one side of the wound. The surrounding skin is first undermined. Using long-acting absorbable monofilament suture material (polydioxanone, 2-0 or 3-0 USP) with a swaged-on needle, a bite is taken through the deep portion of the dermis beginning at the limit of the undermined skin, taking care not to penetrate the epidermis. If the bite has been taken correctly, a dimple will appear externally in the skin. The second bite is taken through the fascia in the wound bed closer to the desired location of the wound edge. As suture is secured, using either a surgeon's knot or a slipknot to mitigate tension, the skin will advance toward the center of the wound.[3] Further walking sutures can be placed at least 2 to 3 cm apart on the same, and if desired the opposing, side of the wound, and several rows may be placed.[6] Because they may interfere with the cutaneous blood supply, the number of walking sutures should be restricted to those necessary to mitigate tension on the wound edges before closure of the subcutaneous tissue and skin. The dimples visible in the epidermis will remodel over several weeks to months. This technique is difficult in patients with a thin dermis, such as Greyhounds and cats.[3]

Stent sutures

Stent sutures are sutures that are preplaced deep in the tissue, away from the skin edges and crossing deep to the wound bed that are used to mitigate only mild tension. They may consist of deep simple interrupted sutures tied over a bolster bandage overlying the incision, or vertical mattress sutures supported by a stent to prevent the suture cutting through the skin. Small stents may cause pressure necrosis of the underlying skin; a Penrose drain or short sections of a red-rubber catheter disperse the tension more evenly. Stent sutures should be removed 3 to 4 days postoperatively once stress relaxation of the skin has occurred.[13] The overtightening of tension-relieving or stent sutures may result in devitalization of the skin.

Specific tension-relieving sutures

Sutures that are designed to relieve tension include vertical mattress, horizontal mattress, far-near-near-far (FNNF), and far-far-near-near (FFNN). These suture patterns are not used commonly and are indicated only in the face of minimal tension, or if the tension is cyclic, for example, concomitant with the movement of a joint. Horizontal mattress sutures are not recommended because they can disrupt the blood supply to the skin edges, and vertical mattress sutures lead to eversion of the wound edges.[3] For FNNF and FFNN suture patterns, the far-far component is placed approximately 1 cm from the incision and provides tension relief.[3] The near component is placed 5 mm from the incision and provides apposition of the skin edges.[3]

Skin-Stretching Techniques

Skin is viscoelastic and has inherent extensibility, the amount of which is dependent on intrinsic factors such as species, individual, location, and age.[17] When placed under tension, skin demonstrates the properties of mechanical creep and stress relaxation.[17] Mechanical creep is the phenomenon where skin elongates when constant tension is applied, because of straightening and realignment of the dermal collagen fibers.[18] Stress relaxation occurs when skin is stretched a set distance and the tension required to keep the skin stretched to that distance decreases over time; that is, the skin loses its tendency to recoil when the load is released.[19]

Presuturing and pretensioning

Although presuturing and pretensioning are both methods of recruiting skin using sutures, presuturing is performed before wound formation (for example, preplanning for a mass excision), whereas pretensioning is used on existing wounds.[3]

For presuturing, large Lembert sutures are placed 3 to 5 cm from the wound edge to imbricate the skin approximately 24 hours before wound closure. Presuturing is a simple technique but is limited regarding the amount of skin that can be recruited and in that the degree of tension cannot be adjusted.[6] For practical purposes, this technique is useful in areas where elastic skin is limited (extremities) and for smaller defects.

Pretensioning can be performed over 24 to 72 hours before closure of a large defect or the development of a local flap. The tissue surrounding the wound must be healthy for pretensioning to be performed. There are several methods of pretensioning: the wound edges can be apposed with a simple continuous or continuous horizontal intradermal running pattern using nonabsorbable monofilament suture material. Each free end of the suture can be passed through a button to distribute pressure and then clamped in a 1 to 2 split-shot fishing weights.[6] The suture can be tightened through both ends at 8- to 24-hour intervals until the skin is apposed.[6,20]

Skin stretchers

Skin stretchers are devices applied externally to recruit skin adjacent to and distant to a wound or before elective surgical procedures. They are most useful in areas where there are large areas of skin that can be mobilized, for example, in the neck and trunk.[17] Skin stretchers are available commercially or can be fabricated in-house.[21,22] The commercial system consists of self-adherent Velcro-covered skin patches that are adhered using cyanoacrylate to shaved skin on either side of the defect, 5 to 10 cm away from the wound edge.[22] Adjustable elastic connecting tapes are used to engage the skin patches and are tightened to reduce tension across the wound edges; these are adjusted every 6 to 8 hours. Sufficient skin is often recruited within 48 hours, although these devices may be maintained up to 96 hours.[17] This device can also be maintained for 2 to 5 days postoperatively to offset incisional tension.[17]

The commercial skin stretcher does not appear effective when used on the lower extremities.[21] Groups of skin staples placed 0.5 cm away from and perpendicular to the skin edges and hypodermic needles passed through the skin edges have been described as effective skin stretchers in experimental closure of skin defects on the limbs of dogs.[21] Undermining of the skin before skin stretching, at least on extremity wounds, does not appear to decrease tension on the wound edges.[21]

Tissue expanders

Tissue expanders are inflatable, expandable, or self-inflating silicone elastomeric bags of predetermined volumes that are placed into a subcutaneous pocket of skin adjacent to a defect. The bag is connected to a silicone tube and a self-sealing injection port. The bag can be inflated rapidly or gradually. Gradual inflation or expansion results in biologic creep, the property of skin where new dermal and epidermal components are created with prolonged constant loading.[3] Expansion results in decreased subcutaneous fat, decreased dermal thickness, and epidermal proliferation, as well as enhanced skin perfusion due to the delay phenomenon.[6,17] The overlying skin is often not as pliable as normal skin due to the fibrous capsule that forms around the expander.

Tissue expanders typically form part of a delayed or staged reconstruction. They are particularly useful for small to moderate defects in the mid to distal extremities.[17] The base of the expander should approximate the size of the donor site. The expander should be inserted through an incision parallel to tension lines at the leading edge of the future flap. Rapid expansion may be performed intraoperatively and involves inflating the expander for 2 to 3 minutes and deflating for 3 to 4 minutes 2 to 3 times before creating a flap.[20] Gradual expansion is performed more commonly; the surgical incision is allowed to heal for several days before expansion of the device by 10% to 15% final volume of sterile saline every 48 to 72 hours until the final volume is achieved.[13] Adding a maintenance period allows for improved quality of the expanded skin. Flap elevation is performed 48 hours after last injection.[17] The incision used to insert the implant should not be incorporated into the base of the flap. Complications may include pain, seroma, infection, dehiscence, implant extrusion, skin necrosis, and implant failure.[17]

Negative pressure wound therapy

Negative pressure wound therapy (NPWT) can be used to recruit skin preoperatively as a skin-stretching device and also over closed surgical incisions to relieve tension and shear forces on the wound edges.[13] A recent case report described the successful use of NPWT to maintain the viability of a rotation flap over the thoracic region.[23] It was reported that NPWT may reduce edema, increase blood flow, and secure the flap onto the recipient bed.[24] (Please see Bryden J. Stanley's article, "Negative Pressure Wound Therapy," in this issue for more information on this technique.)

Tension-Relieving Incisions

Relaxing or releasing incisions are created parallel and adjacent to a wound, allowing the intervening skin to be used to close the primary defect.

Multiple relaxing incisions (mesh expansion)

This technique is most useful to relieve tension in an area where there is limited elasticity of the adjacent skin, for example, the distal extremities, ear, or tail. Circumferential meshing of limb may be performed.[13] Following undermining of the skin, staggered parallel rows of full-thickness stab incisions are made adjacent to the wound. The incisions should be 1 cm long, at least 1 cm from the wound edge, and 1 cm apart.[3] One or more staggered rows may be placed 1 cm apart, depending on the amount of tension. To minimize the number of relaxing incisions made, the skin edges should be under tension using towel clamps, skin or stay sutures while they are being made. A nonadherent, semiocclusive dressing and bandage is applied, and the meshed areas are allowed to heal by second intention.

Single relaxing incision

A single relaxing incision is a form of bipedicle advancement flap. A full-thickness skin incision is created parallel to the long axis of the wound, with the width of the skin bridge approximating the width of the original wound. The incision should be at least as long as the wound and is most effective when up to 1.5 times wound length.[25] The length-to-width ratio should not exceed 4:1 because otherwise the vascular supply to the flap will be compromised.[3] After undermining the bridge of skin between the defect and incision, the primary defect is closed. The relaxing incision can either be closed primarily or allowed to heal by second intention.

A "hidden" intradermal release or relaxing incision has also been described, permitting skin relaxation whilst avoiding additional scarring and wound management.[5] The hidden release incision is created by incising in the same location, but only through the dermis while leaving the epidermis intact.

A V-Y-plasty is a form of relaxing incision that is useful to release a small amount of tension. It is a lengthening procedure useful in revision scars involving the palpebral region and for closure of fusiform defects. A chevron or V-shaped incision is made adjacent to the wound (no closer than 3 cm),[6] with the tip of the "V" facing away from the wound. The skin between the V and wound is undermined and the wound is closed. The incision will have assumed a Y-shaped configuration and is closed beginning at the ends of the arms and ending with the stem.[20]

Z-plasty

Using a Z-plasty, skin can be relocated from one plane into the perpendicular plane to achieve the goal of (1) lengthening restrictive scars, (2) realigning tissues that have healed resulting in distortion of a vital structure or orifice, or (3) reducing tension adjacent to an incision.[26] Incisions in the shape of a "Z" (central limb and 2 arms) are made, resulting in the creation of 2 interdigitating triangular flaps of skin adjacent to a wound. These equilateral triangles can then be transposed, lengthening the skin in the direction of the central limb.

To create a Z-plasty, the central limb incision should be made parallel and over the tension band, in the direction in which relaxation is required, at least 3 cm away from the wound edge.[3] The arms are of equal length to the central limb and are angled back from it at 60°. By transposing the resultant triangular skin flaps, there is a gain in length along the direction of the original central limb, and the central limb changes direction. The net gain in length is the difference between the length of the original central arm (contractural or long diagonal) and the length of a line drawn between the apices of the 2 original arms (transverse or short diagonal).[26]

Effect of arm angle on length gain

The arm angle controls the *percentage* increase in length along the central limb. The greater the arm angle, the greater the net gain in length. A 60° arm angle is recommended; this theoretically gains 75% of the length (clinically closer to 50%).[5] Wider-angle flaps do result in a greater net gain in length; arm angles of 75 to 90° gain 100% and 120% of the central limb length, respectively.[5] However, transposing these flaps is difficult because of the increased tension in the transverse plane. Angles less than 60° result in inadequate lengthening and have narrow flaps, potentially compromising their blood supply.

Effect of limb length on length gain

The limb length controls the *absolute* increase in length along the central limb. Given the arm angle chosen is most often 60°, limb length will have the greatest effect on the length gained. The nature of the surrounding tissue will determine the desired limb length. Although the expected gain in length can be calculated, this often cannot be achieved because of tension or scarring in the surrounding tissue.

The most common complication with Z-plasty is necrosis of the flap tips. Maximum vascular capacity may be achieved by curving the arms away from the central limb so the tips are wider (modified Z-plasty or S-plasty).[26]

LOCAL FLAPS

Local or subdermal plexus flaps are tongues of skin and subcutaneous tissue that are elevated immediately adjacent to and mobilized into the recipient bed, analogous to random or cutaneous flaps in people.[27] They are a practical way to close defects that cannot be closed by the more simple techniques. Local flaps rely on the subdermal plexus entering at the flap base for their vascular supply.[25] Having their own blood supply is an advantage when compared with a skin graft because they can be relocated into areas with poor vascularity. As local flaps are generated from neighboring tissue and the dermis and hypodermis remains intact, they offer excellent long-term durability and cosmesis, being similar in texture, thickness, color, and hair type to the wound bed before wounding.[28] The donor area should have enough loose elastic skin to generate a flap of sufficient size while still being able to be closed without tension or deformation of a vital structure, limiting their use in the lower extremities.

Local flaps are divided into those that rotate or pivot around a point central to their base into position (rotation, transposition, and interpolation) and those that travel in a forward direction with no lateral movement or advancement flaps (single and bipedicle advancement flaps).[28]

Planning a Local Flap

Skin tension and pliability should be assessed by manually lifting or pushing the skin toward the defect.[29] The donor bed should be amenable to primary closure after the flap has been elevated. The shape of the recipient bed should be considered; triangles can often be closed with single or paired rotation flaps, whereas rectangles or squares are often closed with advancement flaps.[27] The length and width of the desired flap should be evaluated. As the subdermal plexus has regional variations, there is no set flap base-to-length ratio. It is recommended that a narrow base be avoided because this could reduce perfusion to the body of the flap and increase the chance of partial necrosis. However, it is important to note that increasing the width at the base of the flap does not necessarily increase the workable viable length.[27] General recommendations are to use a flap with a base slightly wider than the width of the flap body and to limit the length to that required to cover the recipient bed without tension.[27] It is helpful to use a piece of sterile paper drape material to approximate the size and shape of the recipient bed, along with additional skin required to get from the recipient bed to the donor site. The drape is positioned over the defect, and the base is held in a fixed position as the drape is transferred to the donor site to form a final template.[29] The proposed donor site is marked with a marking pen. The flap is often planned slightly larger than the recipient bed to ensure appropriate coverage after transposition; any excess skin can be trimmed before closure. Closure is performed with 1 to 2 subcutaneous layers, followed by cutaneous sutures, staples, or adhesive.[25]

The recipient bed should have been adequately prepared, meaning there should not be any foreign debris, necrotic tissue, or evidence of ongoing infection.[25] Ideally chronic granulation beds should be excised and epithelialized skin edges removed.[27] The flap edges should be secured with interrupted sutures; alternatively, cyanoacrylate adhesive has been described to result in thinner and more aesthetic scars.[15]

Flaps That Rotate About a Pivot Point

Rotation flaps

Rotation flaps are semicircular flaps that share a common border with a triangular defect.[29] They are rotated about a pivot point into the adjacent recipient bed, covering the triangular defect.[27,28] No secondary defect is created because the donor site is closed concomitant to the rotation. Rotation flaps are particularly useful where skin is available on only one side of a lesion or where closure of local skin would distort an orifice for example, eye, anus. A curved incision is made in a stepwise fashion and the flap is undermined until it can cover the wound.[27] A back-cut can be used to relieve tension by allowing the flap to move by transposition and rotation; however, this reduces the vascular area at the base of the flap and should be avoided where possible.[28] Burow triangles can be excised outside and tangent to the circle to relieve tension, although these have been described as only minimally effective.[27,28]

Transposition flaps

Transposition flaps are rectangular pedicle grafts on a different axis to the defect that are elevated and rotated across intact skin into the defect.[28] One edge of the defect is a portion of the flap border. The flap is pivoted between 45° and 90° relative to the long axis of the defect into the recipient site. A 90° transposition flap is aligned parallel to the lines of greatest tension so its donor bed can often be closed easily.[29] The flap can be pivoted greater than 90°; however, the further the arc of rotation, the shorter its effective length. The width of the flap should approximate the width of the defect. The flap must be longer than the defect because there will be a loss of effective length as the flap is rotated. The pivot point is at the far side of the flap's base. To prevent tension, the flap length should approximate the diagonal length from the pivot point at the flap base to the most distant part of the defect. The donor bed is closed primarily. The main disadvantage of transposition flaps is the dog-ear that forms at the base of the flap at the side of the defect after rotation. Removing the dog-ear from this location runs the risk of devascularization of the flap, and therefore, delayed removal (14–21 days) has been described.[28] The vulval fold and surrounding skin were recently described as a specific transposition flap for reconstruction of large perineal defects.[30]

Interpolation flaps

Interpolation flaps are rectangular flaps rotated about a pivot point into a recipient bed that is nearby but not immediately adjacent to the defect; that is, there is no common border with the defect.[25] The pedicle therefore has to pass over or under tissue in between the donor and recipient sites. A bridging incision can be made between the donor and recipient site. Alternatively, the redundant portion of the flap that is overlying the interposing skin is excised 14 days later. Although this flap is not used commonly in veterinary medicine, a specific example is a lip-to-lid flap.[25]

Advancement Flaps

Single-pedicle advancement flaps

A single-pedicle advancement flap is the most simple and commonly used local flap, also referred to as a sliding flap. It consists of skin that is undermined and moved into a defect without altering the plane of the pedicle. Two skin incisions are made progressively, equal to the width of the wound and diverging slightly. The distant skin edge borders the wound and is grasped and elevated so the flap can be undermined. Advancement of the undermined flap results in the closure of both the donor and the recipient beds. Burow triangles may be excised lateral to the base of the flap to equalize the length between the flap and the adjacent wound margins, although these are rarely required. The flap is secured using 3-0 monofilament sutures in the subcuticular layer and skin. The scrotal flap has been described as a specific advancement flap for closure of inguinal and perineal defects.[31]

H-plasty

H-plasty is the formation of 2 shorter single pedicle advancement flaps on either side of a wound.[25] It should be considered when there is loose skin on both sides of a wound because it avoids the use of a single long flap that may be prone to vascular compromise.

Bipedicle advancement flaps

Bipedicle advancement flaps are a form of relaxing incision. They are formed by making an incision parallel to the long axis of the defect, undermining the underlying subcutaneous tissue, and advancing the skin into the defect. Curving the incision with the concave side toward the defect may facilitate advancement.[29] The donor bed is closed by direct apposition after undermining, or it can be left to heal by second intention. These flaps have 2 sources of circulation and can maintain a longer flap body. The flap should approximate the width of the defect and be 2 to 3 times as long as it is wide. The donor site can usually be closed primarily. This closure may be performed on one or both sides of the defect.[27] V-Y advancement is a form of bipedicle advancement flap.

Complications of Local Flaps

Complications reported with local flaps include infection, seroma formation, dehiscence of the wound edges, and flap necrosis.[25] To reduce the incidence of seroma formation, active drains may be placed, along with soft padded bandages and exercise restriction to encourage adherence of the flap to the underlying wound bed.[25] Dehiscence is most often due to excessive tension on the flap edges, although infection or inadequate blood supply may be implicated.[25]

Flap necrosis is often due to technical error such as too narrow a flap base or damage to the subdermal plexus during flap elevation.[25] Other causes include thrombosis, decreased perfusion due to systemic reasons, or self-trauma.[25] Flap necrosis occurs because of a combination of venous congestion and arterial insufficiency, with the arterial component considered more important. Flap viability can be assessed subjectively using color, temperature, and bleeding along the skin margins.[27] Objective methods such as fluorescein dye and laser Doppler blood flow evaluation are not often used clinically. It is not uncommon for flaps to appear congested in the first 24 to 72 hours; true flap necrosis may not become apparent for 5 to 6 days. Partial necrosis of the distant edges of the flap is more common than complete flap necrosis; devitalized skin may undergo liquefactive necrosis or form an eschar.[25]

Attempts at salvaging failing flaps may include hyperbaric oxygen therapy, drug therapy, hirudotherapy (the application of medicinal leeches), and vacuum-assisted closure.[23,32] A small consistent improvement in survival of local flaps has been documented with hyperbaric oxygen therapy.[33] Autologous platelet-rich plasma injected between a long (5:1) subdermal plexus flap and its recipient bed was reported to significantly decrease edema and improve perfusion and survival of flaps in dogs.[34] Leeches are typically reserved for flaps with venous congestion (**Fig. 1**). The saliva of the medicinal leech (*Hirudo medicinalis*) contains hirudin, an anticoagulant that stimulates venous outflow.[35] Recommendations in the human literature include a frequency of application to the compromised area of the flap (typically the distal tip) every 2 to 8 hours for 4 to 10 days.[36] They should be allowed to detach

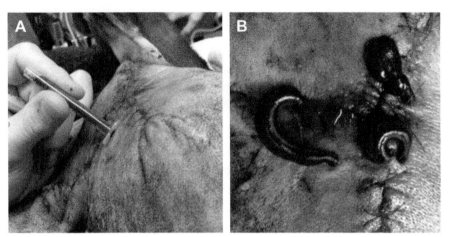

Fig. 1. Application of a leech to a congested rotation flap 24 hours postoperatively (*A*). Three leeches attached to the tip of the congested flap (*B*).

spontaneously once they have finished feeding. There is no consensus as to the number of leeches to use during each application; each leech is thought to increase perfusion in a 2-cm² area. For practical purposes, application of 2 to 5 leeches once a day for 1 to 3 days is used in veterinary patients. Each leech removes 5 to 10 mL of blood during feeding, and leakage of serosanguineous fluid from attachment site occurs for several hours after the leech has detached. In humans, up to 50% of treated patients require a blood transfusion; this does not seem to be a significant concern in veterinary patients likely because of the less intensive treatment protocol. There is a theoretic risk of infection, specifically with *Aeromonas hydrophila*, which may precipitate flap failure (**Fig. 2**); human patients are routinely prescribed antibiotic prophylaxis.[35,36]

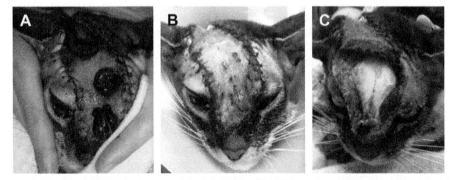

Fig. 2. Leeches attached to a congested rotation flap 24 hours postoperatively (*A*). Focal necrosis of the attachment sites 72 hours postoperatively (*B*). Full-thickness flap necrosis with exposure of the underlying bone 5 days postoperatively (*C*). Exuberant leeching and infection were suspected to have contributed to flap failure. (*Courtesy of* Dr Valery Scharf, DVM, MS, North Carolina State University College of Veterinary Medicine, Raleigh, NC.)

SUMMARY

Successful primary or delayed primary wound closure can often be achieved simply by adhering to basic surgical principles and simple tension-relieving techniques. More advanced tension-relieving techniques can be used preoperatively, intraoperatively, and postoperatively to reduce tension on the skin edges and recruit neighboring skin. Local flaps are useful to close wounds that cannot be closed by the more simple techniques; however, accurate flap planning and meticulous surgical technique are essential to optimize flap viability.

REFERENCES

1. Fahie MA. Primary wound closure. In: Tobias KM, Johnston SA, editors. Veterinary surgery: small animal. St Louis (MO): Elsevier Saunders; 2013. p. 1197–209.
2. Williams J. Decision-making in wound closure. In: Williams J, Moores A, editors. BSAVA manual of canine and feline wound management and reconstruction. 2nd edition. Quedgeley (England): British Small Animal Veterinary Association; 2009. p. 25–36.
3. Stanley BJ. Tension-relieving techniques. In: Tobias KM, Johnston SA, editors. Veterinary surgery: small animal. St Louis (MO): Elsevier Saunders; 2013. p. 1221–42.
4. Waldron DR, Zimmerman-Pope N. Superficial skin wounds. In: Slatter D, editor. Textbook of small animal surgery. 3rd edition. Philadelphia: Saunders; 2003. p. 259–73.
5. Pavletic MM. Tension relieving techniques. In: Pavletic MM, editor. Atlas of small animal wound management and reconstructive surgery. 3rd edition. Ames (IA): Wiley Blackwell; 2010. p. 241–85.
6. Trout NJ. Principles of plastic and reconstructive surgery. In: Slatter D, editor. Textbook of small animal surgery. 3rd edition. Philadelphia: Saunders; 2003. p. 274–92.
7. Swaim S. General principles of delayed wound excision and closure. In: Swaim S, editor. Surgery of traumatized skin: management and reconstruction in the dog and cat. Philadelphia: WB Saunders Company; 1980. p. 237–96.
8. Sylvestre A, Wilson J, Hare J. A comparison of 2 different suture patterns for skin closure of canine ovariohysterectomy. Can Vet J 2002;43:699–702.
9. Swaim S. Moving local tissues to close surface defects. In: Swaim S, editor. Surgery of traumatized skin: management and reconstruction in the dog and cat. Philadelphia: WB Saunders Company; 1980. p. 297–320.
10. Johnston DE. Plastic and reconstructive surgery. Vet Clin North Am 1990;20: 67–80.
11. Irwin DH. Tension lines in the skin of the dog. J Small Anim Pract 1966;7:593–8.
12. Pavletic MM. Skin grafting and reconstruction techniques. In: Bojrab MJ, Waldron DR, Toombs JP, editors. Current techniques in small animal surgery. 5th edition. Jackson (MS): Teton New Media; 2014. p. 595–607.
13. Stanley BJ. Taming tension in wound closure. In: ACVS surgical summit proceedings. 2012. Available at: https://www.acvs.org/files/proceedings/2012/data/papers/122.pdf. Accessed January 10, 2017.
14. Zellner EM, Hedlund CS, Kraus KH, et al. Comparison of tensile strength among simple interrupted, cruciate, intradermal, and subdermal suture patterns for incision closure in ex vivo canine skin specimens. J Am Vet Med Assoc 2016;248: 1377–82.

15. De Carvalho Vasconcellos CH, Matera JM, Zaidan Dagli ML. Clinical evaluation of random skin flaps based on the subdermal plexus secured with sutures or sutures and cyanoacrylate adhesive for reconstructive surgery in dogs. Vet Surg 2005;34:59–63.

16. Swaim SF. A walking suture technique for closure of large skin defects in the dog and cat. J Am Anim Hosp Assoc 1976;12:597.

17. Pavletic MM. Skin-stretching techniques. In: Pavletic MM, editor. Atlas of small animal wound management and reconstructive surgery. 3rd edition. Ames (IA): Wiley Blackwell; 2010. p. 287–305.

18. Melis P, Noorlander ML, van der Horst CMAM, et al. Rapid alignment of collagen fibers in the dermis of undermined and not undermined skin stretched with a skin-stretching device. Plast Reconstr Surg 2002;109:674–80.

19. Wilhelmi BJ, Blackwell SJ, Mancoll JS, et al. Creep vs. stretch: a review of the viscoelastic properties of skin. Ann Plast Surg 1998;41:215–9.

20. Fowler D. Distal limb and paw injuries. Vet Clin North Am Small Anim Pract 2006; 36:819–45.

21. Tsioli V, Papazoglou LG, Papaioannou N, et al. Comparison of three skin-stretching devices for closing skin defects on the limbs of dogs. J Vet Sci 2015;16:99–106.

22. Pavletic MM. Use of an external skin-stretching device for wound closure in dogs and cats. J Am Vet Med Assoc 2000;217:350–4.

23. Bristow PC, Perry KL, Halfacree ZJ, et al. Use of vacuum-assisted closure to maintain viability of a skin flap in a dog. J Am Vet Med Assoc 2013;243:863–8.

24. Krug E, Berg L, Lee C, et al. Evidence-based recommendations for the use of negative pressure wound therapy in traumatic wounds and reconstructive surgery: Steps towards an international consensus. Injury 2011;42(suppl 1):S1–12.

25. Hunt GB. Local or subdermal plexus flaps. In: Tobias KM, Johnston SA, editors. Veterinary surgery: small animal. St Louis (MO): Elsevier Saunders; 2013. p. 1243–55.

26. Swaim S. Z-, V-Y, and W-plasties. In: Swaim S, editor. Surgery of traumatized skin: management and reconstruction in the dog and cat. Philadelphia: WB Saunders Company; 1980. p. 395–422.

27. Pavletic MM. Pedicle Grafts. In: Slatter D, editor. Textbook of small animal surgery. 3rd edition. Philadelphia: Saunders; 2003. p. 292–321.

28. Swaim S. Skin flaps. In: Swaim S, editor. Surgery of traumatized skin: management and reconstruction in the dog and cat. Philadelphia: WB Saunders Company; 1980. p. 321–68.

29. Pavletic MM. Skin flaps in reconstructive surgery. Vet Clin North Am Small Anim Pract 1990;20:81–103.

30. Hunt GB, Winson O, Fuller MC, et al. Pilot study of the suitability of dorsal vulval skin as a transposition flap: vascular anatomic study and clinical application. Vet Surg 2013;42(5):523–8.

31. Matera JM, Tatarunas AC, Fantoni DT, et al. Use of the scrotum as a transposition flap for closure of surgical wounds in three dogs. Vet Surg 2004;33(2):99–101.

32. Buote NJ. The use of medical leeches for venous congestion. Vet Comp Orthop Traumatol 2014;27:173–8.

33. Friedman HI, Friedman HIF, Fitzmaurice M, et al. An evidence-based appraisal of the use of hyperbaric oxygen on flaps and grafts. Plast Reconstr Surg 2006; 117(7 Suppl):175S–90S.

34. Karayannopoulou M, Papazoglou LG, Loukopoulos P, et al. Locally injected autologous platelet-rich plasma enhanced tissue perfusion and improved survival of

long subdermal plexus skin flaps in dogs. Vet Comp Orthop Traumatol 2014;27: 379–86.

35. Welshhans JL, Hom DB. Are leeches effective in local/regional skin flap salvage? Laryngoscope 2016;126:1271–2.

36. Herlin C, Bertheuil N, Bekara F, et al. Leech therapy in flap salvage: systematic review and practical recommendations. Ann Chir Plast Esthet 2017;62: 1–13.

Axial Pattern Flaps

Kelley Thieman Mankin, DVM, MS

KEYWORDS

- Flap • Wound closure • Axial pattern

KEY POINTS

- Axial pattern flaps are useful to close large wounds.
- The vessel that the flap depends on for blood must be viable.
- Axial pattern flaps come in many varieties.
- The most common complication is distal flap necrosis.

INTRODUCTION: NATURE OF THE PROBLEM

Historically, delay procedures were used in reconstructive surgery in order to develop the circulation to sections of skin before transfer.[1] Later, axial pattern flaps were described in veterinary medicine and became an option for closure of large defects without a delay procedure.[2] Axial pattern flaps (APFs) are flaps of skin that incorporate a direct cutaneous artery and vein at their base.[2] Because of the direct cutaneous blood supply, a large area of skin can be transferred acutely. The survival area of flaps with direct cutaneous vessels (APFs) is better than in flaps without direct cutaneous vessels (random pattern flaps). A survival of 95% was reported for flaps with direct cutaneous vessels, whereas a survival area of 53% was reported for flaps without direct vasculature.[1] Other advantages of APF include full thickness, durable skin, excellent cosmetic results, and, in most cases, no need for delay before transposition.

INDICATIONS/CONTRAINDICATIONS

APFs are useful in many circumstances. APFs are used when much skin is needed to fill a defect whether that be following trauma or following removal of a mass. Generally, the recipient site must be a healthy wound free of infection; however, the presence of granulation tissue is not required. Flaps are more cosmetic and robust than free grafts. Therefore, an APF may be chosen over a free graft when durable, full-thickness skin is needed to cover a wound, such as on an extremity of a working dog.

APFs can be used during reconstruction from tumor removal, but several considerations must be taken. First, if clean margins are not attained during mass removal, the

The author has nothing to disclose.
Department of Small Animal Clinical Sciences, College of Veterinary Medicine and Biomedical Sciences, Texas A&M University, College Station, TX, USA
E-mail address: kthieman@cvm.tamu.edu

entire surgical field will be considered seeded with tumor cells. Therefore, a subsequent surgery would require resection of the original tumor site as well as the donor site. For surgeries in which clean margins are questionable, delaying closure of the wound bed may be prudent while awaiting margin analysis. The open wound can be managed with a variety of dressings; this author prefers negative pressure wound therapy (see Bryden J. Stanley's article, "Negative Pressure Wound Therapy," in this issue). Following confirmation of clean resection, the wound can be closed as appropriate.

Whether the APF is used to close a traumatic wound or a surgically created wound, the direct cutaneous vessels supplying the APF must be viable.

TECHNIQUE/PROCEDURE
Preparation

In some animals, the viability of the direct cutaneous vessel may be in question, either because the mass excision encroached on the origin of the vessel or because of trauma or injury to the surrounding soft tissues. Identifying the vessel preoperatively can be performed with Doppler flow ultrasound or by using an ultrasonic Doppler flow detector. One study evaluated the ability of ultrasound and color flow Doppler ultrasound to assess direct cutaneous vessels used for APFs in dogs.[3] They evaluated 4 direct cutaneous vessels: the superficial cervical, thoracodorsal, deep circumflex iliac, and caudal superficial epigastric arteries.[3] The study concluded that a combination of fundamental ultrasonographic and color flow Doppler ultrasonographic imaging is easy and noninvasive and can be used to identify the 4 direct cutaneous vessels commonly used for APFs in dogs.[3] They suggested that this method of identification may be useful in planning APFs, especially in dogs that have experienced trauma and the viability of the direct cutaneous vessel is in question.[3]

APF development requires careful planning in order to optimize outcome. Measuring the defect and drawing the margins of the flap on the animal preoperatively or intraoperatively minimizes errors. Rotating the flap into its new position leads to a shortened flap and a dog ear created at the point of rotation. Shortening should be taken into account when planning the APF. APFs can be rotated up to 180° at the base in order to cover the defect. Rotation greater than 180° may cause venous occlusion, resulting in venous congestion and flap necrosis.

Skin stretchers may be used to elongate the skin preoperatively.[4] A case report has been published on preoperative skin stretching to elongate a thoracodorsal APF for an antebrachial wound closure. In the case report, the skin over the scapula was stretched using adhesive pads and elastic cables. The preoperative skin stretching provided an estimated 8 to 10 cm of additional skin for reconstruction.[4]

Patient Positioning

Patient positioning depends on the location of the wound and on which APF is planned to be used for closure. The skin must be in a neutral position when planning the APF. Anatomic landmarks are used to delineate the flap margins. If the skin is pulled one way or another, the angiosome may be shifted, causing distortion with respect to anatomic landmarks and possibly resulting in flap failure. Generally, the limbs are placed in a natural, relaxed position and the skin is lifted and allowed to spontaneous retract to its natural position.[5]

APPROACH
Technique/Procedure

The animal is prepared in routine fashion, including a wide clip of surrounding fur. The amount of skin needed in the surgical field is easy to underestimate, so clipping wider than expected is important to allow some flexibility in the surgical plan and to allow space to close the donor site.

In animals with chronic wounds, several millimeters of healing edges may be removed from the recipient site in order to provide fresh, bleeding skin to which the flap can be sutured.

The landmarks and surgical recommendations for many common APF are detailed later. All APFs should be elevated deep to the cutaneous trunci muscle or equivalent. This position provides as little disruption to the vascular supply as possible during elevation. Elevation commences at the distal tip of the skin flap and proceeds toward the base. Gentle handling of the flap is facilitated by placement of stay sutures in the distal flap, rather than manipulation with thumb forceps.

After elevating an APF, the skin can be rotated into the defect. The donor site is closed routinely and may require elevation and walking sutures. Once the APF is rotated into its new position, the subcutaneous tissue is sutured with a small-diameter, absorbable suture in an interrupted or continuous suture pattern. The corners can be tacked down first to assess the ability of the flap to fill the defect, and then the remainder is sutured. No sutures are necessary in the middle of the APF as sutures may inadvertently puncture and damage the direct cutaneous vessel. Therefore, dead space is expected under the APF. Some surgeons will elect to place a closed suction drain to prevent seroma formation. After the subcutaneous tissues are closed, the skin is closed with staples or skin sutures.

APFs come in either a peninsula or island form. The peninsula APF maintains a cutaneous attachment at its base. An island APF is created by dividing the cutaneous pedicle but preserving the underlying direct cutaneous artery and vein. An island flap has more mobility and is helpful when the original wound encroaches up on the origin of the direct cutaneous artery and vein. Islandizing a flap is not recommended for some flaps as detailed later.

Caudal superficial epigastric

The caudal superficial epigastric APF is a versatile, robust, useful flap. The flap can be used to close skin defects of the caudal abdomen, flank, inguinal area, prepuce, perineum, thigh, and rear limbs.[2] The flap includes the caudal 3 or 4 mammary glands. Mammary gland function remains unchanged after flap relocation, and an ovariohysterectomy can be considered. The animal is placed in dorsal recumbence. The medial incision begins caudal to the last mammary teat and proceeds cranially on the ventral midline, including the last 3 to 4 mammary glands. In male dogs, the midline of the flap must hug the prepuce in order to incorporate the vasculature. The flap is planned to be as short as possible to cover the wound but may extend to end between glands 1 and 2 or 2 and 3.[2] The lateral incision is developed parallel to the medial incision. The lateral incision should be the same distance from the mammary teats as the medial incision. Once the incision is completed, the flap is undermined just superficial to the abdominal fascia.[2]

Genicular

The genicular APF is useful in closing skin wounds of the lateral or medial tibial region.[2] Depending on the confirmation of the dog, the flap may have the ability to extend distally to the level of the tibiotarsal joint. The animal is positioned in lateral recumbency. The flap is marked at a point 1 cm proximal to the patella and 1.5 cm below the tibial tuberosity. The two lines are extended on the lateral thigh parallel to the shaft of the femur proximally to the greater trochanter. The flap is elevated by undermining and then rotated into the lower limb defect.[2]

Omocervical/superficial cervical

The omocervical APF is useful in closing large skin defects involving the face, head, ear, shoulder, neck, and axilla.[2,6] The animal is positioned in lateral recumbence. The forelimb is placed in relaxed extension perpendicular to the trunk. The caudal margin of the flap is the spine of the scapula. The cranial shoulder depression is palpated and the distance measured between the caudal margin and the cranial shoulder depression. The cranial margin of the flap is parallel to the caudal margin and an equal distance cranial to the cranial shoulder depression as the caudal margin is caudal to the cranial shoulder depression. The length of the flap can extend as far as the contralateral scapulohumeral joint but is reliably extended to dorsal midline.[2,6] In cats, the flap can be more reliably extended to the contralateral scapulohumeral joint.[6] The extension of the flap to the contralateral shoulder is essential if the flap is to be used for reconstruction of the face or dorsal head.[6] This flap has been termed the extended superficial cervical APF and has been used to repair large oral defects caudal to the third premolar spanning 50% to 75% of the width of the palate by passing the flap through a parapharyngeal tunnel.[7]

Thoracodorsal

The thoracodorsal APF is useful in closing skin wounds of the shoulder, forelimb, elbow, axilla, and thorax.[2] The animal is placed in lateral recumbence. The forelimb is placed in relaxed extension perpendicular to the trunk. The cranial margin of the flap is the spine of the scapula. The distance between the cranial margin and the caudal shoulder depression (at the level of the acromion process) is measured. The caudal margin of the flap is parallel to the cranial margin and placed so that the cranial and caudal margins are equal distances from the caudal shoulder depression.[2] The length of the flap can extend as far as the contralateral scapulohumeral joint.

Superficial brachial

The superficial brachial APF is useful in closing skin wounds of the antebrachium and elbow. This APF is based on a small cutaneous vessel and meticulous surgical technique is important. The animal is placed in dorsal recumbence. The entire limb is prepared for surgery. The base of the flap is centered over the anterior third of the flexor surface of the elbow.[2] The lateral and medial borders are formed parallel to each other extending proximally, parallel to the humeral shaft. The medial and lateral borders should be gradually converging tapering the proximal portion of the flap. The lines are connected at or below the proximal point of the greater tubercle.[2] This flap can be especially helpful when used as an island APF when the wound of the antebrachium abuts the origin/base of the superficial brachial APF (**Fig. 1**).

Deep circumflex iliac (dorsal and ventral)

The deep circumflex iliac APF comes as a dorsal or ventral form based on either the dorsal or ventral branch of the deep circumflex iliac artery and vein. The dorsal branch is useful for closing skin wounds of the ipsilateral flank, lateral lumbar area, caudal thorax, lateral thigh, and pelvic area.[2] The animal is positioned in lateral recumbence. The hind limb is in relaxed extension perpendicular to the trunk. The vessel exits the lateral abdominal wall just cranio-ventral to the wing of the ilium and proceed dorsally. The

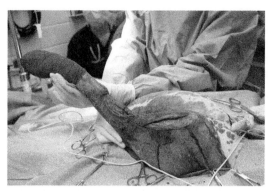

Fig. 1. Superficial brachial APFs.

base of the flap is centered over this vessel. The caudal margin of the flap is midway between the cranial border of the wing of the ilium and the greater trochanter.[2] The cranial margin is parallel to the caudal incision and equal to the distance between the iliac border and caudal margin.[2] The incisions proceed dorsally and conclude at dorsal midline.[5]

The ventral branch may be most useful as an island arterial flap for closure of sacral and lateral pelvic skin wounds. Again, the animal is positioned in lateral recumbence. The landmarks for the width of the flap are the same as with the dorsal branch, but this vessel proceeds ventrally. The caudal margin begins at the midpoint between the wing of the ilium and greater trochanter and is directed distally, cranial to the border of the femoral shaft. The cranial margin extends from the established point cranial to the wing of the ilium down the flank and parallel to the caudal flap margin. The flap ends proximal to the patella by connecting the cranial and caudal margins.[2] A variation on the ventral deep circumflex APF is the flank fold flap. This flap can be used to close frustrating wounds in the inguinal area. For this variation, a U-shaped incision is made after grasping loose tissue available on the cranial aspect of the thigh. The limb must be put through a range of motion in order to plan appropriately to avoid excessive tension when closing the donor site.[5]

Reverse saphenous conduit

The reverse saphenous conduit APF is useful for closing skin wounds at or below the tarsus, especially over the metatarsal surface.[2] When extensive trauma has occurred to the limb, the saphenous artery and medial saphenous vein should be assessed preoperatively in order to determine their viability and the remaining blood supply to the distal limb. The animal is positioned in dorsal recumbence. The entire limb is prepared. A skin incision is made across the central third of the medial limb at or slightly proximal to the patella. Scissors are used to expose the underlying saphenous artery, medial saphenous vein, and nerve. Two incisions are extended proximally and converging slightly. The two incisions are positioned 0.5 to 1.0 cm cranial and caudal to the borders of the cranial and caudal branches of the saphenous artery and medial saphenous vein, respectively.[2] The flap is undermined deep to the vasculature. A portion of the medial gastrocnemius muscle fascia is included with the flap. The tibial nerve merges with the descending caudal branches of the saphenous artery and medial saphenous vein and can be preserved by careful dissection between the two structures. Ligation and division of the peroneal (fibular) artery and vein are needed to provide mobility of the flap.[2,8]

Caudal auricular

The caudal auricular APF is useful to close wounds of the face, neck, dorsal head, and ear. The animal is placed in lateral recumbence or as appropriate for the wound closure. Inconsistent survival of the distal flap is common.[6] The base of the flap is the depression between the wing of the atlas and the vertical ear canal at the base of the ear. The width of the flap varies. In dogs, it is the central third of the lateral cervical region over the wing of the atlas. In cats, the dorsal incision is on dorsal midline. The distance between the depression and the dorsal incision is measured, and the ventral incision is placed an equal distance ventral to the depression and parallel to the dorsal incision. The flap can be extended to the spine of the scapula.[8] This flap is not amenable to being developed as an island flap; instead, bridging incisions should be used if needed to place the flap on the face or head.[6] Single-stage, bilateral use of this flap is likely impossible because of the skin tension when closing the donor site at the neck (**Fig. 2**).

Superficial temporal

The superficial temporal APF is useful to close wounds of the cheek, lip, periorbital region, and caudal aspect of the bridge of the nose, palate, and medial eyelid.[6,8] The flap should be elevated deep to the frontalis muscle as the vessel runs within the muscle. The caudal margin of the flap is a line across the forehead rostral to the ear. The rostral margin runs parallel to the caudal orbital border. The width of the flap is approximately equal to the length of the zygomatic arch with the caudal orbital rim as the rostral border and the caudal zygomatic arch as the caudal border. The flap length can be up to the middle of the contralateral eye.[5,6] This flap performs better as a peninsula flap and should not be made into an island flap.[6] Additionally, distal flap necrosis is common when the flap is extended to its full length. For that reason, it is suggested that the flap not exceed a 3:1 length-to-width ratio.[6]

Cranial cutaneous branch of saphenous

The cranial cutaneous branch of the saphenous APF is a recently described APF. Descriptions of this APF were based on cadaveric perfusion studies, and no clinical information is published. This APF could be used to close wounds on the cranial distal thigh and stifle, the popliteal region, and the proximal medial crus.[9] Landmarks for creation of this flap include the cranial border of the thigh to the level of the saphenous vessels caudally. Proximodistal margins include the level of the medial condyle distally and extending proximally to two-thirds the distance to the inguinal ring.[9] This flap is

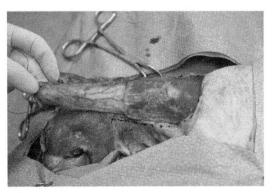

Fig. 2. Caudal auricular APFs.

not amenable to creation of an island APF and instead should be a peninsula in order to allow closure of the donor site.[9]

Lateral caudal (tail)

The lateral caudal APF is useful to close wounds in the perineum or caudodorsal pelvic area. The animal is placed in dorsal or sternal recumbence, as appropriate. The first incision is on the dorsal or ventral midline of the tail depending on whether the wound to be closed with the flap is located dorsally or ventrally, respectively. The skin is dissected free of the bone preserving the right and left caudal arteries and veins. The bony part of the tail is amputated at the caudal second-third intervertebral space.[10] The length of the flap can extend to the tip of the tail if necessary; but the most useful area is the thicker, proximal third of the tail. If placed ventrally, the flap can be split along the distal midline so that each half has a blood supply and each half can cover the respective side of the anus[10] (**Fig. 3**).

Cutaneous branch of the dorsal perineal artery

An APF based on the cutaneous branch of the dorsal perineal artery has been described in a cat. This flap was used to close a defect on the proximal third of the tail and may provide an alternative to tail amputation for animals requiring mass removal or wound closure on the tail. The medial and lateral landmarks used for flap elevation were the medial and lateral aspects of the ischiorectal fossa. The medial and lateral incisions were parallel to each other and extended ventrally for approximately 8 cm. The base of the flap was 3 cm. The published report could not establish safe borders; but they theorized that if perfusion studies were performed, the flap could be even larger than that elevated in this report.[11]

Facial artery/angularis oris

An APF based on the angularis oris artery, branches of the facial artery, in both dogs and cats has been described. This flap is useful in reconstructing large facial, nasal, and chin defects.[12,13] The base of the skin flap is centered on the commissure of the lip and extends caudodorsally. The dorsal and ventral margins are the ventral aspect of the zygomatic arch and the ventral aspect of the horizontal mandibular ramus, respectively. The dorsal and ventral incisions are made parallel to each other and extending caudodorsally to the vertical ear canal or as far as the

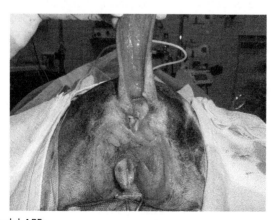

Fig. 3. Lateral caudal APFs.

wing of the atlas depending on the length needed. The flap is raised in a caudal to rostral direction, but rostral dissection is limited.[12,13] Transillumination has been suggested to verify the presence of the target vessels.[13] This flap can also be used following maxillectomy but results in billowing of the flap due to air motion.[12] A similar flap has been described in cats as a perfusion study.[14] The borders in the cat were determined to be as follows: Rostral is a dorsoventral line that passes through the rostral edge of the masseter muscle. The ventral border is ventral midline and extends from the rostral border to a point 1 cm caudal to the wing of the atlas. The caudal border is a dorsoventral line on the neck passing 1 cm caudal to the caudal border of the wing of the atlas. The dorsal border is a line parallel to the ventral border at a distance from the origin similar to the distance from the origin to the ventral border, which is approximately 1 cm ventral to the zygomatic arch.[14]

A variation of the angularis oris APF has been described to raise a buccal mucosal flap for reconstruction of palatal lesions following tumor resection or recurrent oronasal fistulas.[15,16] This buccal flap is raised by palpating a pulse just caudal to the commissure of the lips. The skin is not moved in this flap, just buccal mucosa. A skin incision is made over the artery starting at the commissure of the lips and extending caudally. The skin is reflected in order to see the angularis oris artery and vein. Identification of the vessels can be facilitated by using transillumination of the cheek tissue. After the vessel is identified, the subcutaneous tissue, buccal tissue, and oral mucosa are transected dorsal and ventral to the vessels and extending caudally to the caudal extent of the buccal pouch. The flap can be islandized to allow greater mobility.[16] Survival of this flap may be improved by preprocedural removal of teeth that are likely to cause occlusal trauma to the flap's pedicle.[17]

COMPLICATIONS AND MANAGEMENT

Overall, the survival rate of APFs is high. When partial flap failure occurs, it is typically necrosis of the distal tip of the flap. The most common causes of flap necrosis are inadequate blood supply and infection. Inadequate blood supply can be caused in several ways. Complete arterial or venous obstruction can occur if the vessel was missed during elevation of the flap, if sutures were inadvertently placed through or around the vessels at the base of the flap, or if the vessels were compromised or thrombosed because of excessive rotation/manipulation of the pedicle. Excessive wound tension can also result in decreased blood supply to the flap. Experimentally, a hematoma underlying the flap can lead to flap death because of pressure generated beneath the flap leading to vascular compromise or because of the hemolysate itself.[8]

A study was performed evaluating the tolerance of cutaneous and mucosal flaps placed in to radiation therapy fields.[18] The study included all cutaneous or mucosal flaps (advancement flaps, transposition flaps, and APFs). The study revealed an overall 77% complication rate. The study looked at 3 different groups: animals undergoing a flap procedure at the time of tumor removal followed by radiation therapy, animals undergoing radiation therapy followed by surgery and flap procedure, and, finally, animals undergoing a flap procedure in order to treat complications associated with previously performed radiation therapy. The reported complication rates for each group were 55.6%, 87.5%, and 88.9%, respectively, with the most common complication being dehiscence. Although the complication rates were high, flaps were used successfully in a radiation therapy field in 85% of the dogs. The group concluded that flaps can be considered for use in dogs that may undergo radiation therapy.[18]

Different studies evaluated the complications and outcome of the caudal superficial epigastric APF and the thoracodorsal APF for reconstruction of skin - defects in dogs.[19,20] In each study, the investigators evaluated 10 dogs that had undergone wound closure with either a caudal superficial epigastric APF or a thoracodorsal APF for hind or front limb wounds, respectively. Considering the dogs who had wounds closed with the caudal superficial APF, 3 developed seromas, 3 developed partial dehiscence (small segment), and 9 developed edema. Overall, 9 dogs had complete flap survival. The one dog that experienced some flap necrosis had had an external fixator pin placed through the APF. The total area of survival for all 10 dogs was estimated at 99.96%. The most common complication was bruising and edema of the distal flap, and the investigators suspected venous and lymphatic compromise caused the bruising and edema. The study also reported that dogs that had undergone trauma as the reason for the APF being performed stayed in the hospital longer than dogs undergoing APF for closure of a wound after tumor removal (11.0 days vs 2.7 days for tumor removal). No long-term complications were reported. The other study assessed the complications and outcome of the thoracodorsal APF.[20] The findings were surprisingly different in that only 3 of the 10 dogs had complete flap survival.

POSTOPERATIVE CARE

Postoperative analgesia is important. A multimodal approach is recommended. Icing the flap is not recommended. Many surgeons place a bandage over the flap and donor site to apply some gentle compression and help reduce dead space and serve as a barrier to bacterial contamination. When bandages are placed, care must be taken to avoid excessive compression, which could lead to tissue damage.

To aid in survival, many anecdotes are suggested. Literature is sparse with regard to the amount of benefit that can be attained using various methods. Leech therapy has been suggested in order to facilitate venous drainage when venous congestion occurs (**Fig. 4**).

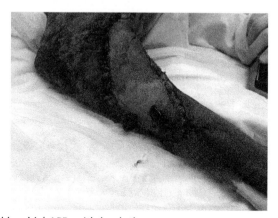

Fig. 4. Superficial brachial APFs with leech therapy.

SUMMARY

APFs are useful to close large wounds. The vessel that the flap depends on for blood must be viable at the start and at the end of surgery. APFs come in many varieties. The most common complication is distal flap necrosis.

REFERENCES

1. Pavletic MM. Canine axial pattern flaps, using the omocervical, thoracodorsal, and deep circumflex iliac direct cutaneous arteries. Am J Vet Res 1981;42:391.
2. Pavletic MM. Axial pattern flaps in small animal practice. Vet Clin North Am 1990; 20:105–25.
3. Reetz JA, Seiler G, Mayhew PD, et al. Ultrasonographic and color-flow Doppler ultrasonographic assessment of direct cutaneous arteries used for axial pattern skin flaps in dogs. J Am Vet Med Assoc 2006;228:1361–5.
4. Holt DE, Runge J. Use of skin stretchers to elongate a peninsular thoracodorsal axial pattern flap for antebrachial wound closure in a dog. Vet Surg 2011;40: 352–6.
5. Pavletic MM. Axial pattern skin flaps. In: Pavletic MM, editor. Atlas of small animal wound management & reconstructive surgery. 3rd edition. Ames (IA): Wiley-Blackwell; 2010. p. 357–401.
6. Degner DA. Facial reconstructive surgery. Clin Tech Small Anim Pract 2007;22: 82–8.
7. Dundas JM, Fowler JD, Shmon CL, et al. Modification of the superficial cervical axial pattern skin flap for oral reconstruction. Vet Surg 2005;34:206–13.
8. Wardlaw JL, Lanz OI. Axial pattern and myocutaneous flaps. In: Tobias K, Johnston S, editors. Veterinary surgery small animal. St Louis (MO): Elsevier Saunders; 2012. p. 1256–70.
9. Murdoch AP, Greenaway SN, Owen LJ, et al. Evaluation of an axial pattern flap based on the cranial cutaneous branch of the saphenous artery: a cadaveric perfusion study. Vet Surg 2016;45:922–8.
10. Saifzadeh S, Hobbenaghi R, Noorabadi M. Axial pattern flap based on the lateral caudal arteries of the tail in the dog: an experimental study. Vet Surg 2005;34: 509–13.
11. Murdoch AP, Grand JGR. An axial pattern flap based on the dorsal perineal artery in a cat. Aust Vet J 2016;94:470–3.
12. Yates G, Landon B, Edwards G. Investigating and clinical application of a novel axial pattern flap for nasal and facial reconstruction in the dog. Aust Vet J 2007; 85:113–8.
13. Losinski SL, Stanley BJ, Schallberger SP, et al. Versatility of the angularis oris axial pattern flap for facial reconstruction. Vet Surg 2015;44:930–8.
14. Milgram J, Weiser M, Kelmer E, et al. Axial pattern flap based on a cutaneous branch of the facial artery in cats. Vet Surg 2011;40:347–51.
15. Dicks N, Boston S. The use of an angularis oris axial pattern flap in a dog after resection of a multilobular osteochondroma of the hard palate. Can Vet J 2010; 51:1274–8.
16. Bryant KJ, Moore K, McAnulty JF. Angularis oris axial pattern buccal flap for reconstruction of recurrent fistulae of the palate. Vet Surg 2003;32:113–9.
17. Cook DA, Thompson MJ. Complications of the angularis oris axial pattern buccal flap for reconstruction of palatine defects in two dogs. Aust Vet J 2014;92:156–60.
18. Seguin B, McDonald DE, Kent MS, et al. Tolerance of cutaneous or mucosal flaps placed into a radiation therapy field in dogs. Vet Surg 2005;34:214–22.

19. Aper RL, Smeak DD. Clinical evaluation of caudal superficial epigastric axial pattern flap reconstruction of skin defects in 10 dogs (1989-2001). J Am Anim Hosp Assoc 2005;41:185–92.
20. Aper R, Smeak D. Complications and outcome after thoracodorsal axial pattern flap reconstruction of forelimb skin defects in 10 dogs, 1989-2001. Vet Surg 2003;32:378–84.

Free Grafts and Microvascular Anastomoses

Valery F. Scharf, DVM, MS

KEYWORDS

- Free grafts • Free skin flaps • Microvascular anastomoses • Wounds • Engraftment

KEY POINTS

- Skin grafts are classified by their morphology and source and rely on healthy vascularity of the recipient bed.
- Engraftment or "graft take" is the process of integration of the graft and consists of adherence, plasmatic imbibition, inosculation, and vascular ingrowth.
- Free skin flaps are developed from described axial pattern flaps and use microvascular anastomoses to reattach the flap's direct cutaneous vessels to recipient vessels near a distant wound.
- Skin grafts and free skin flaps are useful ways of closing wounds in which local flaps or primary closure are not feasible, such as distal extremity defects or large wounds on the trunk.
- Successful engraftment requires careful atraumatic technique, proper recipient bed preparation, and diligent postoperative monitoring and bandaging.

INTRODUCTION

Veterinary surgeons are occasionally presented with wounds that cannot be closed primarily or with local or axial pattern flaps. These are most frequently wounds located on the distal extremities beyond the reach of available local flaps, although alternative methods of closure also may be required in wounds that are too extensive to be closed with local tissue. Several techniques for grafting distant skin have been extrapolated from human plastic surgery to address such wounds, and additional free grafts have been developed and described in the veterinary literature.[1–3]

Unlike axial pattern flaps, free grafts rely entirely on the development of arterial and venous connections developing with the recipient bed. The process of engraftment, or graft "take," can be divided into 4 general phases: adherence, plasmatic imbibition,

Disclosure Statement: The author has nothing to disclose.
Small Animal Soft Tissue Surgery, Department of Clinical Sciences, North Carolina State University College of Veterinary Medicine, 1060 William Moore Drive, Raleigh, NC 27606, USA
E-mail address: vfscharf@ncsu.edu

inosculation, and vascular ingrowth. Adherence begins immediately following graft placement, as fibrin strands link collagen and elastin on the graft and recipient bed. The first and second phase of adherence involve the polymerization of fibrin strands followed by conversion to fibrous adhesions, leading to an increase in strength that occurs until a fibrous union occurs by approximately 10 days postoperatively.[1,4–8]

Plasmatic imbibition is the process whereby graft vessels dilate and absorb serum-like fluid and cells into the graft vessels. Imbibition is responsible for nourishing the graft until vasculature is established. The graft typically has a purple or cyanotic appearance during this time, with edema peaking at 48 to 72 hours postoperatively.[1] The third phase of engraftment, inosculation, is the anastomosis of vessels from the graft with those of the recipient bed, usually occurring between 48 and 72 hours after graft placement. The graft generally begins to be perfused by the third or fourth day after grafting, with blood flow reaching normal velocity by the fifth or sixth day.[9]

New vessels also grow into the graft from the recipient bed through the process of vascular ingrowth, which occurs at a rate of 0.5 mm/d and peaks at days 5 to 7 after grafting.[1,10] New lymphatic vessels also begin forming by day 4 or 5 after grafting. Reinnervation is greater in full-thickness grafts compared with split-thickness grafts and is influenced by additional factors such as type of graft and surrounding tissue. A successful graft is generally fully healed by approximately 3 weeks after grafting.[1]

INDICATIONS/CONTRAINDICATIONS

Skin grafts are indicated for wounds in which mobilization of surrounding skin or local flaps is insufficient for coverage of the wound. The most common location for free grafts is the distal limbs in which loose skin is sparse and available flaps are limited, although grafts are also frequently used to cover large skin defects over the trunk.

Several factors contribute to graft failure and as such there are many contraindications to free grafts. In addition to systemic contraindications, such as anemia, cachexia, uremia, hypoperfusion, and other systemic disease leading to chronic inflammation, local contraindications include infection and a high-motion wound bed.[1] Whenever possible, measures should be taken to address systemic and local factors before grafting (eg, culture-based antimicrobial therapy for infection, blood transfusion for anemia); other tactics may be adopted postoperatively to address local factors (ie, splinting for high-motion areas).

Free grafts require a vascularized wound bed for successful grafting, thus a graft recipient site must contain viable muscle, periosteum, peritenon, or granulation tissue. A graft must be placed either over healthy granulation tissue or a clean, vascular, acute wound. In dogs, studies have shown that grafts over fresh tissue have faster vascularization than grafts placed over granulation tissue.[11,12] As grafts require vascular ingrowth from the underlying bed, grafting over surfaces lacking good vascular supply (bone, cartilage, tendon, avascular fat, or heavily irradiated tissues) is not recommended. Similarly, grafting over hypertrophic or chronic granulation tissue is also contraindicated due to excessive inflammation and poor vascularity, respectively.[1]

Free grafts are classified according to source, thickness, and shape. Autografts, in which the graft is harvested from the recipient, are the main type of graft used in veterinary medicine, as opposed to allografts (homografts, or grafts from a different animal of the same species) and xenografts (heterografts, or grafts from an animal of a different species). Split-thickness or partial-thickness grafts consist of epidermis and a varying partial amount of dermis, whereas full-thickness grafts consist of the entire epidermis and dermis. Both split-thickness and full-thickness grafts can be applied as meshed or unmeshed grafts. The advantages and disadvantages of different graft conformations are listed in **Table 1**. Due to their thin skin, split-thickness grafts are not recommended in cats.[1]

TECHNIQUE/PROCEDURE
Preparation

Before grafting, careful consideration must be given to the type of graft to be harvested as well as to the location and method of closure of the donor site. The ideal donor site has similar coloration and hair growth to the recipient site and enough neighboring loose skin that it can be closed primarily if desired. Additionally, thinner skin is more likely to have successful vascular ingrowth and graft "take." For these reasons, the cranial lower thoracic area is the most common donor site in companion animals.[1] A morphometric analysis of different donor sites in dogs found that mean epidermal and dermal thickness of the dorsal lumbar and lateral neck regions were greater than those of other regions, making these sites less ideal for graft harvest.[13] The dorsal lumbar region had the highest hair follicle density, and hair follicle density in the prepared full-thickness grafts was significantly lower than in intact skin specimens, indicating that even full-thickness grafts may have reduced hair density compared with neighboring skin.[13]

Positioning

Patient positioning must be planned carefully. Ideally, the patient should be positioned in such a way that the graft can be both harvested and placed in the recipient bed

Table 1
Advantages and disadvantages of different skin graft techniques

Graft Type	Advantages	Disadvantages
Full-thickness	• Improved cosmesis • Superior hair regrowth • Improved durability	• Decreased engraftment
Split-thickness	• Improved engraftment • Donor bed may heal via adnexal regeneration and epithelialization	• Contraindicated in cats • Less durable • Poorer cosmesis • More susceptible to secondary graft contraction • Requires specialized equipment
Meshed	• Improved drainage • Improved conformity • Improved expansion	• Excess granulation tissue • Poorer cosmesis
Unmeshed	• Minimal postgraft contraction • Superior hair regrowth and cosmesis	• Increased risk of fluid accumulation or infection, leading to graft failure
Partial coverage or "seed" grafts (pinch, punch, strip, and stamp)	• May be used on contaminated wounds • May be used on irregular wounds • Rapid engraftment • Easy donor site closure • May induce contraction and epithelialization	• Require granulation tissue at recipient site • Less durable • Poor cosmesis

without repositioning the patient. If this is not possible, the graft should be kept moist in moistened gauze sponges while the donor site is closed, the patient repositioned, and the recipient site prepared. Graft storage via refrigeration has been described in humans and horses but is not routinely indicated in small animals.[2]

Technique/Procedure

Graft bed preparation
Before grafting, the recipient bed should be free of infection and prepared to receive the graft to minimize risk of graft failure. Granulation tissue should be healthy and fresh to maximize vascular ingrowth. In surgery, the superficial granulation tissue may be lightly scraped with a scalpel blade or gently wiped with a gauze sponge. A #15 scalpel blade is used to freshen the edges of the surrounding skin by removing epithelial cells from the wound edge. The wound is then covered with a gauze sponge soaked in 0.05% chlorhexidine diacetate in saline or 0.25% neomycin in saline while the graft is harvested.[1]

Graft harvest
After the recipient bed is prepared, a tracing of the wound is made using sterile paper drape. This tracing is transferred to the donor site, maintaining the correct orientation to the skin's surface, and adjusting the template such that the direction of hair growth at the donor site will match the direction of hair growth surrounding the recipient site. The tracing is then outlined on the donor site. For full-thickness grafts, a scalpel blade is used to cut the outline of the graft, and the graft is sharply dissected using Metzenbaum scissors. Some surgeons prefer to cut the graft approximately 1 cm wider than the outline of the recipient site. The graft should be handled delicately, with skin hooks used to apply gentle traction to the graft as needed.

Split-thickness grafts are often harvested using a specialized graft knife. There are several types of graft knives available, including the Weck knife (a Goulian-type graft knife with a fixed guard and disposable blade), and the Humby and Watson knives with adjustable guards. For knives with adjustable guards, the depth is ideally set at 0.35 mm for dogs, which is approximately equal to the width of a #10 blade handle.[1,7] A dermatome is a power-driven tool with an oscillating blade that can alternatively be used to harvest split-thickness grafts. Sterile saline is injected subcutaneously at the donor site to elevate the skin, which is then lubricated with a sterile lubricant to facilitate the use of the dermatome. Partial-thickness grafts also may be harvested using a razor or scalpel blade by hand, although this is more tedious and challenging than using a specialized graft knife or dermatome.

Graft preparation
Full-thickness grafts are "defatted" by stretching flat over the surgeon's index finger or affixing dermal-side-up to a sterile surface, such as a piece of cardboard using hypodermic needles at the corners of the graft to maintain tension (**Figs. 1** and **2**). While keeping the graft moistened with sterile saline or lactated Ringer's solution, all of the subcutaneous tissue is removed using sharp, delicate scissors. All subcutaneous tissue should be removed until the dermis has the characteristic cobblestone appearance from the exposed bulbs of hair follicles. Mesh grafts are meshed by using a #11 blade to cut parallel rows of 1-cm to 2-cm incisions staggered approximately 0.5 to 2 cm apart or by using a mesh graft expansion unit.[14]

Graft placement
Once prepared, the graft is placed over the recipient bed and sutured to the edge of the wound in a simple interrupted or cruciate pattern, or using skin staples.[7] Some

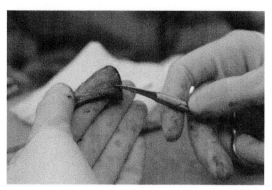

Fig. 1. Preparation of a full-thickness free graft using tenotomy scissors to "defat" the graft, removing subcutaneous tissue until the bulbs of hair follicles are visible. The scissors point to the characteristic cobblestone appearance of the exposed hair follicles.

surgeons prefer to suture the edges of the graft directly the edges of skin surrounding the recipient bed; others suture the graft to the defect leaving 0.5 to 1.0 cm of graft overlapping the skin surrounding the recipient bed. The overlapping graft edges will ultimately necrose and can be trimmed as the graft heals.[7] Mesh grafts may be slightly expanded by trimming an additional 2 to 3 mm of skin from the free edge of the graft before it is sutured. Additional simple interrupted sutures between edges of some slits and the underlying recipient bed are placed to further secure the graft to the wound. These sutures should be placed sparingly to avoid excessive trauma to the graft; sites should be chosen to maximize contact between the graft and the underlying wound bed (**Fig. 3**). Occasional simple interrupted sutures also may be placed in the center of unmeshed grafts to bring the central portion of the graft in close contact with the underlying wound bed.

Island grafts
Various types of seed or island grafts are harvested and placed in a similar manner. Punch grafts are harvested using a 4-mm-diameter skin punch biopsy, whereas strip grafts are harvested as 5-mm-wide strips that are placed in 2-mm-deep grooves approximately 3 to 5 mm apart.[1] Stamp grafts may be harvested as either partial-thickness or full-thickness squares. Seed grafts are placed on granulation tissue

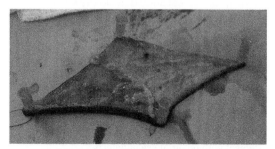

Fig. 2. A partially prepared full-thickness free graft in which the subcutaneous tissue has been removed from the right half of the graft, creating a characteristic cobblestone appearance of the bulbs of hair follicles. The graft is pinned to a sterile plastic surface using 25-gauge hypodermic needles to facilitate preparation.

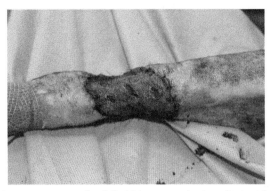

Fig. 3. Postoperative appearance of a full-thickness meshed graft over the distal crus. Note the minimal use of sutures in the center of the graft to minimize trauma to the graft.

beds, and their security can be improved by creating pockets or grooves in the recipient granulation tissue depending on the shape of the graft. Pockets 2 to 4 mm in depth are made approximately 5 to 7 mm apart for pinch grafts and 1 to 2 cm apart for punch grafts, in a staggered fashion.[1] Hemorrhage from the recipient sites can be controlled via manual pressure. Excessive hemorrhage should be avoided, as it can further separate the graft from the underlying wound bed and prevent graft take.

Donor sites may be closed primarily or left to heal by second intention; primary closure is preferred, as it avoids additional bandaging and wound care. Occasionally, donor sites may be closed with the use of local flaps.

Other grafts
The following site-specific grafts have been described for various uses:

- Paw pad grafts are small full-thickness segments of pad tissue placed on recipient beds of granulation tissue over an absent metacarpal or metatarsal pad.[1]
- Scrotal free grafts may be used as full-thickness meshed grafts to treat distal limb degloving injuries in dogs.[3]
- Mucosal grafts may be harvested from buccal or sublingual mucosa for various uses (**Box 1**).[1] Mucosal grafts may be meshed or unmeshed, and underlying muscle and submucosa should be removed with delicate scissors before grafting. Planning of the graft harvest should avoid the sublingual vessels and salivary duct, and donor sites are closed with 3 to 0 or 4 to 0 absorbable monofilament suture.[1]

Box 1
Applications of mucosal grafts

- Replacement of nictitans membrane
- Mucosal lining for preputial reconstruction
- Conjunctival replacement with repair of eyelid defects
- Lining reconstructed nasal passages
- Urethroplasty

COMPLICATIONS AND MANAGEMENT

Complications are frequent with free grafts, with survival rates of 58% to 89% historically reported for full-thickness and partial-thickness grafts, respectively.[15] Partial-thickness grafts are reported to have improved survival compared with full-thickness grafts, although more recent literature and the author's experience suggest that full-thickness grafts may achieve equivalent engraftment to partial-thickness grafts with proper preparation.[2,16,17] Common causes of graft failure include accumulation of fluid (seroma or hematoma) between the graft and wound bed, shearing forces from movement, and infection.[18] Fluid accumulation beneath the graft can be mitigated via use of a meshed graft or placement of a closed suction drain beneath the graft.[7] The benefits of drainage must be weighed against the potential disruption caused by placing a drain between the wound bed and the overlying graft.

For nonacute wounds or those in which contamination is suspected, the recipient wound bed should be cultured before graft placement so that susceptibility-guided antimicrobial therapy can be initiated for wounds in which contamination is a concern. Some surgeons prefer to place all graft patients on systemic broad-spectrum antibiotics before surgery and postoperatively for 1 week.[2] The recipient bed should be thoroughly cleaned in surgery with a 1:40 chlorhexidine-saline or chlorhexidine lactated Ringer solution, and triple antibiotic ointment should be generously applied to the surface of the graft postoperatively to further minimize risk of infection.[2] Postoperative movement and disruption of the graft can be minimized with bandaging, immobilization of the affected limb through splinting, and activity restriction.

The use of negative pressure wound therapy (NPWT) has gained prominence as a useful adjunct for promoting graft survival in humans and dogs.[17,19–25] NPWT is thought to improve wound healing through increased blood flow to the wound, increased granulation tissue formation, decreased interstitial edema, and improved bacterial clearance.[26–31] The theoretic improvement in immobilization and the removal of fluid from beneath meshed grafts is theorized to further contribute to the positive effects of NPWT on engraftment.[17] An experimental study of full-thickness meshed grafts on the antebrachia of dogs found that granulation tissue appeared earlier in grafts treated with NPWT, and percent graft necrosis and remaining open mesh area were both reduced in NPWT-treated grafts compared with control grafts at most time points.[17] For use of NPWT over grafted wounds, the author prefers to cover the graft with a single-layer petrolatum-impregnated knitted cellulose-acetate dressing as the primary layer. An open-cell foam with pores of 400 to 600 μm is then placed over the dressing and secured with a plastic adhesive dressing overlapping the wound edges by several centimeters to create a seal. Depending on the location of the wound, a modified Robert Jones bandage is placed over the adhesive dressing such that the suction tubing exits the bandage to connect to the vacuum device. This outer bandage provides additional protection and immobilization and can incorporate a splint if indicated. Pressure is set at −65 to −75 mm Hg in a continuous or intermittent setting and maintained for a minimum of 2 to 4 days postoperatively.[1,17,18]

POSTOPERATIVE CARE

Careful postoperative management is critical to successful grafting. With few exceptions, grafts should be bandaged postoperatively to protect the graft from trauma and contamination and to help maintain contact between the graft and the recipient bed. Antibiotic ointment should be placed gently around the edges of the graft and along the surface of a nonadherent dressing, which is then placed against the graft. A modified Robert Jones bandage is then placed over the nonadherent dressing. Tie-over bandages also may be used for wounds over the trunk or in areas not amenable to modified Robert Jones bandages. Alternatively, the graft can be covered with a foam dressing and attached to a vacuum-assisted device to apply negative pressure to the graft.[1,2,7,17]

To minimize contamination and trauma to the graft, bandages should be changed as infrequently as possible, with the first change ideally occurring 48 to 96 hours postoperatively, although earlier changes may be necessary due to strike-through, infection, or traumatization of the bandage. Warm saline may be gently poured over the nonadherent dressing as the bandage is removed to prevent the graft from adhering to the contact layer of the bandage. Wounds over joints or in areas of high motion on the limbs should have splints placed within the bandage to immobilize the limb and minimize graft movement. Grafts are generally bandaged for at least 14 to 21 days postoperatively, with splints maintained for 10 to 14 days postoperatively. Continued light bandaging is recommended by some investigators for an additional 1 to 2 weeks after the initial 3-week healing period,[1,7] because, although a study in rats showed reinnervation along the graft margins at 13 days postoperatively, complete reinnervation requires 40 days.[1] Thus, during this time, patients may experience paraesthesia or dysesthesia that may lead to self-traumatization of the graft if left unprotected.

OUTCOMES

The viability of a graft may be assessed by monitoring its appearance. Grafts are initially pale in color and gradually become purple to red during the inosculation phase. By 3 to 4 days postoperatively, the graft becomes a lighter red and should be red to pink by day 7 to 8 (**Figs. 4–6**). A white or pale tan color indicates avascular necrosis, whereas ischemic necrosis can appear as a blackened area (**Fig. 7**).[1] Partial-thickness necrosis may be debrided or allowed to slough, leaving behind dermis that will reepithelialize.

Although free grafts are not as robust as axial pattern flaps, their versatility for use in locations not amenable to skin flaps makes them a valuable tool for closing wounds on the limb or large wounds on the trunk. Partial-thickness grafts are thought to have higher rates of successful engraftment, although more recent studies suggest that full-thickness grafts may have equivalent outcomes.[2,15–17,25] Necrosis may range from partial and superficial (requiring minimal debridement and revision) to full-thickness and complete loss of the grafted skin. Although complete loss of the graft

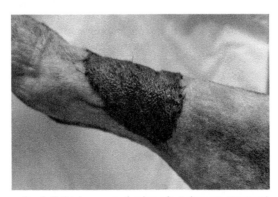

Fig. 4. Appearance of a full-thickness meshed graft 4 days postoperatively. Note the dark red to purple color characteristic of inosculation.

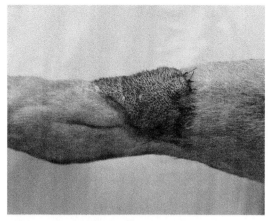

Fig. 5. Appearance of the same graft 2 weeks postoperatively. The graft has developed a light pink appearance and contraction has caused the distal edge of the graft to retract slightly from the edge of the wound bed. This area, along with the open mesh holes, are healing via second intention while the graft continues to be bandaged with triple antibiotic ointment and a nonadherent dressing.

is rare, owners should be prepared for potential graft failure and the need for revision. More commonly, partial necrosis may be managed with debridement and second-intention healing or delayed primary closure of the remaining defect.

FREE FLAP TRANSFER VIA MICROVASCULAR ANASTOMOSES
Indications/Contraindications

Free flap transfer is a hybrid procedure combining the versatility of a free graft with the robust vascular supply of an axial pattern flap, allowing larger flaps to be placed over recipient beds with less than ideal vascularity. This application involves the detachment of axial pattern flaps to distant sites where the direct cutaneous vessels of the flap are microscopically anastomosed to vasculature near the distant wound bed.

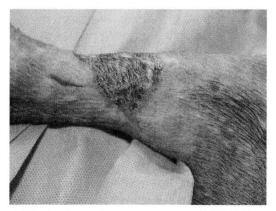

Fig. 6. Appearance of the healed graft 3 weeks postoperatively. Note that the open mesh holes have healed by second intention and the direction of hair growth does not align perfectly with the direction of hair growth on the surrounding skin.

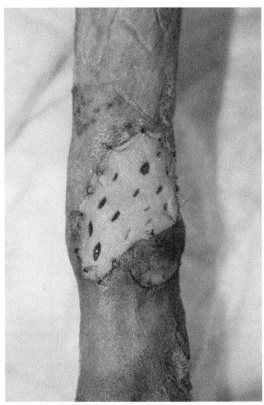

Fig. 7. A full-thickness meshed graft applied to the palmar carpal surface 3 days postoperatively, following removal of NPWT. The diffuse white color of the graft indicates avascular necrosis and complete graft failure. A culture of the wound bed was positive for bacterial growth, suggesting infection as the cause of graft failure.

Free flap transfers require the use of specialized instruments for microsurgery, including the use of an operating microscope for smaller vessels. Due to their improved vascular supply compared with traditional free grafts, free flaps are particularly useful for slow-healing wounds, such as those caused by radiation, chemical or thermal injury, or decubital ulcers.[32]

Technique/Procedure

Five criteria are required for successful transfer of a free skin flap (**Box 2**).[32] Microvascular anastomosis of vessels smaller than 3 mm in diameter requires the use of an operating microscope, with most work performed between ×2 and ×45.[32] Monofilament, nonabsorbable suture, such as nylon or polypropylene, is commonly used, with 9 to 0 suture used for vessels 2 to 3 mm in diameter, and size 10 to 0 used for vessel diameters smaller than 2 mm.[32] Microvascular instruments, including an approximating vascular clamp, atraumatic single vessel clamps, microscissors, nonlocking fine needle drivers, and 2 to 3 jeweler's forceps also should be available.[32]

Any described axial pattern flap may serve as the donor site in the dog. In addition, a free muscular flap using the rectus abdominis muscle has been used experimentally and clinically.[33,34] Described recipient sites in the dog are listed in **Table 2**.[32,35]

Box 2
Criteria required for successful transfer of a free skin flap

1. Adequate size and esthetics

2. Minimal donor site morbidity

3. Consistent vascular pedicle

4. Vascular diameter of $\geq$0.5 mm

5. Vascular pedicle length of $\geq$4.0 cm

As the flap is elevated, initial isolation of the vessel should be performed using loupes with ×4.5 magnification, whereas final identification and isolation should be completed using the operating microscope. Vessel clamps are applied to the isolated vascular pedicle, and the vessels are ligated proximal to the clamps.[32] The recipient site is prepared in a manner similar to that described for free grafts and should be performed by a second surgical team at the same time that the skin flap is being harvested to minimize flap ischemic time.[32] An end-to-end technique is performed between donor and recipient vessels outside the "zone of trauma," with the more

---

Table 2
Described recipient vessels for microvascular anastomoses of free skin flaps

Region	Artery	Vein
Palmar forelimb	Palmar common digital II	Cephalic
Distal antebrachium	Median	Cephalic
Mid-antebrachium	Median	Cephalic
Proximal antebrachium	Median	Cephalic vein, brachial
Distal brachium	Brachial	Brachial
Mid-brachium	Recurrent ulnar	Recurrent ulnar
Plantar hindlimb	Plantar metatarsal	Medial branch of dorsal common digital
Dorsal tarsus	Dorsal pedal	Dorsal common digital or branch thereof
Cranial distal crus	Cranial tibial	Cranial branch of medial saphenous
Craniomedial distal crus	Cranial tibial	Cranial branch of medial saphenous
Lateral distal crus	Saphenous	Lateral saphenous
Caudomedial distal crus	Caudal branch of saphenous	Caudal or cranial branch of medial saphenous
Medial stifle	Saphenous	Medial saphenous
Lateral distal thigh	Distal caudal femoral	Distal caudal femoral
Medial thigh	Femoral	Femoral
Medial proximal thigh	Proximal caudal femoral	Proximal caudal femoral
Groin	Caudal superficial epigastric	Caudal superficial epigastric
Proximal lateral thigh	Caudal gluteal	Caudal gluteal

Data from Degner DA, Walshaw R, David Fowler J, et al. Surgical approaches to recipient vessels of the fore- and hindlimbs for microvascular free tissue transfer in dogs. Vet Surg 2005;34(4):297–309.

difficult end-to-side anastomosis used when vessels are of unequal size. Simple inter-rupted sutures are placed between 2 to 3 initial full-thickness stay sutures, at which time clamps are removed and additional sutures are placed as needed for leaks.[32]

Complications and Management

Free flaps depend on their reperfused direct cutaneous vessel entirely for at least 8 to 14 days postoperatively; thus, these flaps often either survive or show complete fail-ure.[32,36,37] To minimize the risk of thrombosis of the anastomosed vessels, vessel ends are lavaged with 1% to 2% lidocaine to prevent spasm and are flushed with hep-arinized saline immediately before anastomosis. Additionally, some surgeons prefer to administer antiplatelet medication, such as acetylsalicylic acid for several days post-operatively.[32] The average primary critical ischemia time for skin is the time between the severing of the flap's vascular pedicle and its reperfusion at the recipient site at which 50% of flaps survive if reperfused. The secondary critical ischemia time refers to a second ischemic insult that may occur with postoperative complications.[32] These times are 13.0 hours and 7.2 hours, respectively, and if length of ischemia surpasses the critical ischemia times, the flap will fail even when eventually reperfused.[36] Thus, it is critical to minimize ischemic time intraoperatively and to promptly address any post-operative complications.[32] Postoperative care is similar to that of axial pattern flaps, with special attention paid to patient positioning to minimize the risk of vascular compromise.

Outcomes

A retrospective review of 57 free flaps with microvascular anastomoses performed for various causes found a flap survival rate of 93%.[38] In addition to vascular failure, several flaps developed partial dehiscence or wound infection. Flaps were performed for a variety of reasons, and most were performed using an end-to-end technique with either standard suture or an anastomotic coupling device. For flaps in which throm-bosis was noted at the anastomosis or venous flow appeared sluggish intraopera-tively, the original anastomosis was resected and a second anastomosis performed, and all of these flaps ultimately survived. Of the 4 flaps that failed from vascular compromise postoperatively, 3 of the 4 failures were attributed to venous compro-mise, emphasizing the importance of postoperative positioning and care in preventing compression or kinking of the flap's vasculature.[38] Flap failure was directly related to the level of experience of the assistant surgeon, highlighting the importance of expe-rience with microsurgical techniques in the success of performing microvascular free tissue transfer.[38] Microvascular transfer of the rectus abdominis muscle has also been described to successfully cover distant defects, including a resected elbow hygroma in a dog.[34]

SUMMARY

Skin grafts and free skin flaps are useful methods for closure of wounds in which pri-mary closure or the use of skin flaps is not feasible. Grafts are classified by their morphology and by their host-donor relationship. Although partial-thickness skin grafts may demonstrate improved engraftment, full-thickness grafts provide superior durability and cosmesis. Free skin flaps with microvascular anastomoses are devel-oped from previously described axial pattern flaps and have the added advantage of reestablishing robust vascular supply to the flap, but require specialized equipment and a high degree of technical expertise. For either procedure, recipient site prepara-tion and diligent postoperative management are critical for success. Health of the flap may be assessed by physical appearance, and infection, fluid accumulation, physical disruption, and vascular compromise should be addressed immediately. Owners should be prepared for extensive postoperative bandaging and the potential for partial or complete graft or flap failure. Despite these risks and intensive perioperative care, skin grafts and free skin flaps, when performed properly, can provide rewarding methods of closing challenging wounds.

REFERENCES

1. Bohling MW, Swaim SF. Skin grafts. In: Tobias KM, Johnston SA, editors. Veterinary surgery small animal. 1st edition. St Louis (MO): Elsevier Saunders; 2012. p. 1271–90.
2. Pavletic MM. Atlas of small animal wound management & reconstructive surgery. 2nd edition. Ames (IA): Wiley-Blackwell; 2010.
3. Harris J, Dhupa S. Treatment of degloving injuries with autogenous full thickness mesh scrotal free grafts. Vet Comp Orthop Traumatol 2008;21(4):378–81.
4. Grabb WC. Basic techniques of plastic surgery. In: Smith JW, Aston SJ, editors. Grabb and Smith's plastic surgery. 4th edition. Boston: Little, Brown; 1991. p. 3.
5. Swaim SF. Surgery of traumatized skin: management and reconstruction in the dog and cat. Philadelphia: Saunders; 1980.
6. Pope ER. Skin grafting in small animal surgery. Compend Contin Educ Pract Vet 1988;10:915.
7. Swaim SF. Skin grafts. Vet Clin North Am Small Anim Pract 1990;20(1):147–75.
8. Tavis MJ, Thornton JW, Harney JH, et al. Graft adherence to de-epithelialized surfaces: a comparative study. Ann Surg 1976;184(5):594–600.
9. Converse JM, Smahel J, Ballantyne DLJ, et al. Inosculation of vessels of skin graft and host bed: a fortuitous encounter. Br J Plast Surg 1975;28(4):274–82.
10. Most D, Efron DT, Shi HP, et al. Differential cytokine expression in skin graft healing in inducible nitric oxide synthase knockout mice. Plast Reconstr Surg 2001; 108(5):1251–9.
11. Bauer MS, Pope ER. The effects of skin graft thickness on graft viability and change in original graft area in dogs. Vet Surg 1986;15(4):321–4.
12. Jensen EC. Canine autogenous skin grafting. Am J Vet Res 1959;20:898–908.
13. Bhandal J, Langohr IM, Degner DA, et al. Histomorphometric analysis and regional variations of full thickness skin grafts in dogs. Vet Surg 2012;41(4): 448–54.
14. Pope ER. Mesh skin grafting. Vet Clin North Am Small Anim Pract 1990;20(1): 177–87.
15. McKeever PJ, Braden TD. Comparison of full- and partial-thickness autogenous skin transplantation in dogs: a pilot study. Am J Vet Res 1978;39(10):1706–9.
16. Tong T, Simpson DJ. Free skin grafts for immediate wound coverage following tumour resection from the canine distal limb. J Small Anim Pract 2012;53(9): 520–5.
17. Stanley BJ, Pitt KA, Weder CD, et al. Effects of negative pressure wound therapy on healing of free full-thickness skin grafts in dogs. Vet Surg 2013;42(5):511–22.
18. Browne EZJ. Complications of skin grafts and pedicle flaps. Hand Clin 1986;2(2): 353–9.
19. Blackburn JH, Boemi L, Hall WW, et al. Negative-pressure dressings as a bolster for skin grafts. Ann Plast Surg 1998;40(5):453–7.
20. Chang KP, Tsai CC, Lin TM, et al. An alternative dressing for skin graft immobilization: negative pressure dressing. Burns 2001;27(8):839–42.

21. Llanos S, Danilla S, Barraza C, et al. Effectiveness of negative pressure closure in the integration of split thickness skin grafts: a randomized, double-masked, controlled trial. Ann Surg 2006;244(5):700–5.
22. Moisidis E, Heath T, Boorer C, et al. A prospective, blinded, randomized, controlled clinical trial of topical negative pressure use in skin grafting. Plast Reconstr Surg 2004;114(4):917–22.
23. Scherer LA, Shiver S, Chang M, et al. The vacuum assisted closure device: a method of securing skin grafts and improving graft survival. Arch Surg 2002; 137(8):930–4.
24. Landau AG, Hudson DA, Adams K, et al. Full-thickness skin grafts: maximizing graft take using negative pressure dressings to prepare the graft bed. Ann Plast Surg 2008;60(6):661–6.
25. Ben-Amotz R, Lanz OI, Miller JM, et al. The use of vacuum-assisted closure therapy for the treatment of distal extremity wounds in 15 dogs. Vet Surg 2007;36(7): 684–90.
26. Morykwas MJ, Faler BJ, Pearce DJ, et al. Effects of varying levels of subatmospheric pressure on the rate of granulation tissue formation in experimental wounds in swine. Ann Plast Surg 2001;47(5):547–51.
27. Morykwas MJ, Argenta LC, Shelton-Brown EI, et al. Vacuum-assisted closure: a new method for wound control and treatment: animal studies and basic foundation. Ann Plast Surg 1997;38(6):553–62.
28. Morykwas MJ, Simpson J, Punger K, et al. Vacuum-assisted closure: state of basic research and physiologic foundation. Plast Reconstr Surg 2006;117: 121S–6S.
29. Scherer SS, Pietramaggiori G, Mathews JC, et al. The mechanism of action of the vacuum-assisted closure device. Plast Reconstr Surg 2008;122(3):786–97.
30. Weston C. The science behind topical negative pressure therapy. Acta Chir Belg 2010;110(1):19–27.
31. Braakenburg A, Obdeijn MC, Feitz R, et al. The clinical efficacy and cost effectiveness of the vacuum-assisted closure technique in the management of acute and chronic wounds: a randomized controlled trial. Plast Reconstr Surg 2006; 118(2):390–400.
32. Miller CW. Free skin flap transfer by microvascular anastomosis. Vet Clin North Am Small Anim Pract 1990;20(1):189–99.
33. Calfee EF, Lanz OI, Degner DA, et al. Microvascular free tissue transfer of the rectus abdominis muscle in dogs. Vet Surg 2002;31(1):32–43.
34. Green ML, Miller JM, Lanz OI. Surgical treatment of an elbow hygroma utilizing microvascular free muscle transfer in a Newfoundland. J Am Anim Hosp Assoc 2008;44(4):218–23.
35. Degner DA, Walshaw R, David Fowler J, et al. Surgical approaches to recipient vessels of the fore- and hindlimbs for microvascular free tissue transfer in dogs. Vet Surg 2005;34(4):297–309.
36. Kerrigan CL, Zelt RG, Daniel RK. Secondary critical ischemia time of experimental skin flaps. Plast Reconstr Surg 1984;74(4):522–6.
37. Harrison DH, Girling M, Mott G. Experience in monitoring the circulation in free-flap transfers. Plast Reconstr Surg 1981;68(4):543–55.
38. Fowler JD, Degner DA, Walshaw R, et al. Microvascular free tissue transfer: results in 57 consecutive cases. Vet Surg 1998;27(5):406–12.

UNITED STATES POSTAL SERVICE® Statement of Ownership, Management, and Circulation (All Periodicals Publications Except Requester Publications)

1. Publication Title	2. Publication Number		3. Filing Date
VETERINARY CLINICS OF NORTH AMERICA-SMALL ANIMAL PRACTICE	003 – 150		9/18/2017

4. Issue Frequency	5. Number of Issues Published Annually	6. Annual Subscription Price
JAN, MAR, MAY, JUL, SEP, NOV	6	$319.00

7. Complete Mailing Address of Known Office of Publication (Not printer) (Street, city, county, state, and ZIP+4®)

ELSEVIER INC.
230 Park Avenue, Suite 800
New York, NY 10169

Contact Person
STEPHEN R. BUSHING

Telephone (Include area code)
215-239-3688

8. Complete Mailing Address of Headquarters or General Business Office of Publisher (Not printer)

ELSEVIER INC.
230 Park Avenue, Suite 800
New York, NY 10169

9. Full Names and Complete Mailing Addresses of Publisher, Editor, and Managing Editor (Do not leave blank)

Publisher (Name and complete mailing address)

ADRIANNE BRIGIDO, ELSEVIER INC.
1600 JOHN F KENNEDY BLVD. SUITE 1800
PHILADELPHIA, PA 19103-2899

Editor (Name and complete mailing address)

COLLEEN DIETZLER, ELSEVIER INC.
1600 JOHN F KENNEDY BLVD. SUITE 1800
PHILADELPHIA, PA 19103-2899

Managing Editor (Name and complete mailing address)

PATRICK MANLEY, ELSEVIER INC.
1600 JOHN F KENNEDY BLVD. SUITE 1800
PHILADELPHIA, PA 19103-2899

10. Owner (Do not leave blank. If the publication is owned by a corporation, give the name and address of the corporation immediately followed by the names and addresses of all stockholders owning or holding 1 percent or more of the total amount of stock. If not owned by a corporation, give the names and addresses of the individual owners. If owned by a partnership or other unincorporated firm, give its name and address as well as those of each individual owner. If the publication is published by a nonprofit organization, give its name and address.)

Full Name	Complete Mailing Address
WHOLLY OWNED SUBSIDIARY OF REED/ELSEVIER, US HOLDINGS	1600 JOHN F KENNEDY BLVD. SUITE 1800 PHILADELPHIA, PA 19103-2899

11. Known Bondholders, Mortgagees, and Other Security Holders Owning or Holding 1 Percent or More of Total Amount of Bonds, Mortgages, or Other Securities. If none, check box. ▶ ☐ None

Full Name	Complete Mailing Address
N/A	

12. Tax Status (For completion by nonprofit organizations authorized to mail at nonprofit rates) (Check one)
The purpose, function, and nonprofit status of this organization and the exempt status for federal income tax purposes:
☒ Has Not Changed During Preceding 12 Months
☐ Has Changed During Preceding 12 Months (Publisher must submit explanation of change with this statement)

13. Publication Title	14. Issue Date for Circulation Data Below
VETERINARY CLINICS OF NORTH AMERICA: SMALL ANIMAL PRACTICE	JULY 2017

15. Extent and Nature of Circulation			Average No. Copies Each Issue During Preceding 12 Months	No. Copies of Single Issue Published Nearest to Filing Date
a. Total Number of Copies (Net press run)			947	811
b. Paid Circulation (By Mail and Outside the Mail)	(1)	Mailed Outside-County Paid Subscriptions Stated on PS Form 3541 (Include paid distribution above nominal rate, advertiser's proof copies, and exchange copies)	555	495
	(2)	Mailed In-County Paid Subscriptions Stated on PS Form 3541 (Include paid distribution above nominal rate, advertiser's proof copies, and exchange copies)	0	0
	(3)	Paid Distribution Outside the Mails Including Sales Through Dealers and Carriers, Street Vendors, Counter Sales, and Other Paid Distribution Outside USPS®	204	193
	(4)	Paid Distribution by Other Classes of Mail Through the USPS (e.g. First-Class Mail®)	0	0
c. Total Paid Distribution (Sum of 15b (1), (2), (3), and (4))		▶	759	688
d. Free or Nominal Rate Distribution (By Mail and Outside the Mail)	(1)	Free or Nominal Rate Outside-County Copies included on PS Form 3541	99	123
	(2)	Free or Nominal Rate In-County Copies Included on PS Form 3541	0	0
	(3)	Free or Nominal Rate Copies Mailed at Other Classes Through the USPS (e.g. First-Class Mail)	0	0
	(4)	Free or Nominal Rate Distribution Outside the Mail (Carriers or other means)	0	0
e. Total Free or Nominal Rate Distribution (Sum of 15d (1), (2), (3) and (4))		▶	99	123
f. Total Distribution (Sum of 15c and 15e)		▶	858	811
g. Copies not Distributed (See Instructions to Publishers #4 (page #3))		▶	89	0
h. Total (Sum of 15f and g)		▶	947	811
i. Percent Paid (15c divided by 15f times 100)		▶	88.46%	84.83%

* If you are claiming electronic copies, go to line 16 on page 3. If you are not claiming electronic copies, skip to line 17 on page 3.

16. Electronic Copy Circulation		Average No. Copies Each Issue During Preceding 12 Months	No. Copies of Single Issue Published Nearest to Filing Date
a. Paid Electronic Copies	▶	0	0
b. Total Paid Print Copies (Line 15c) + Paid Electronic Copies (Line 16a)	▶	759	688
c. Total Print Distribution (Line 15f) + Paid Electronic Copies (Line 16a)	▶	858	811
d. Percent Paid (Both Print & Electronic Copies) (16b divided by 16c × 100)	▶	88.46%	84.83%

☒ I certify that 50% of all my distributed copies (electronic and print) are paid above a nominal price.

17. Publication of Statement of Ownership

☒ If the publication is a general publication, publication of this statement is required. Will be printed in the NOVEMBER 2017 issue of this publication. ☐ Publication not required.

18. Signature and Title of Editor, Publisher, Business Manager, or Owner

STEPHEN R. BUSHING - INVENTORY DISTRIBUTION CONTROL MANAGER

Stephen R. Bushing

Date 9/18/2017

I certify that all information furnished on this form is true and complete. I understand that anyone who furnishes false or misleading information on this form or who omits material or information requested on the form may be subject to criminal sanctions (including fines and imprisonment) and/or civil sanctions (including civil penalties).

PS Form **3526**, July 2014 (Page 3 of 4)

PS Form **3526**, July 2014 (Page 1 of 4 (see instructions page 4)) PSN: 7530-01-000-9931 PRIVACY NOTICE: See our privacy policy on www.usps.com

PRIVACY NOTICE: See our privacy policy on www.usps.com

Printed and bound by CPI Group (UK) Ltd, Croydon, CR0 4YY

03/10/2024

01040397-0011